OTITIS EXT
– AN ESSENTIAL GUIDE TO
DIAGNOSIS AND TREATMENT

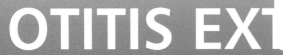

Richard G. Harvey

BVSc, DVD, Dip.ECVD, FSB, PhD, MRCVS
The Veterinary Centre
Cheylesmore, Coventry, UK

Sue Paterson

MA, VetMB, DVD, DipECVD, MRCVS
RCVS and European Specialist in Veterinary Dermatology
Rutland House Referral Hospital
St Helens, Merseyside, UK

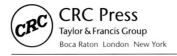

CRC Press
Taylor & Francis Group
Boca Raton London New York

CRC Press is an imprint of the
Taylor & Francis Group, an **informa** business

First published in paperback 2024

First published 2014 by CRC Press

Published 2019 by CRC Press
4 Park Square, Milton Park, Abingdon, Oxon, OX14 4RN

and by CRC Press
2385 NW Executive Center Drive, Suite 320, Boca Raton FL 33431

Publisher's Note
The publisher has gone to great lengths to ensure the quality of this reprint but points out that some imperfections in the original copies may be apparent.

Library of Congress Cataloging-in-Publication Data

Harvey, Richard G., author.
  Otitis externa : an essential guide to diagnosis and treatment / authors, Richard G. Harvey, Sue Paterson.
  p. ; cm.
  Includes bibliographical references and index.
  Summary: "The investigation and management of ear disease occupies a significant proportion of veterinary clinicians time. Otitis externa, in particular, is likely to be seen by busy small animal clinicians at least once a day. Chronic, and chronic recurrent, otitis externa is frustrating, and costly, to the owner and often painful for the dog or cat. This book provides a comprehensive source of information on the relevant structure, function, medicine, and surgery of the ear, from infection to infection, by way of atopy"--Provided by publisher.
  ISBN 978-1-4822-2457-3 (alk. paper)
  I. Paterson, Sue, author. II. Title.
  [DNLM. 1. Ear Diseases--veterinary. 2. Otitis Externa--veterinary. 3. Cat Diseases. 4. Dog Diseases. SF 891]

SF991
636.089'78--dc23   2014006004

ISBN: 978-1-4822-2457-3 (hbk)
ISBN: 978-1-03-283675-1 (pbk)
ISBN: 978-0-429-09508-5 (ebk)

DOI: 10.1201/b16788

Visit the Taylor & Francis Web site at
http://www.taylorandfrancis.com

and the CRC Press Web site at
http://www.crcpress.com

CONTENTS

PREFACE

The investigation and management of ear disease will occupy a significant proportion of a veterinary clinician's time. Otitis externa, in particular, is likely to be seen by a busy small animal clinician at least once a day. Chronic, and chronic recurrent, otitis externa is frustrating and costly to the owner and often painful for the dog or cat.

The concept behind this book is to provide a comprehensive source of information on the relevant structure, function, medicine, and surgery of the ear, from *Otodectes cynotis* infection to *Pseudomonas aeruginosa* infection, by way of atopy.

We hope that students and clinicians, in particular, will find it so useful that their copy becomes battered and stained, the ultimate test of practical relevance.

ABBREVIATIONS

BAER	brainstem auditory evoked response
CT	computed tomography
DMSO	dimethylsulfoxide
EDTA	ethylenediamine tetra-acetic acid
GABA	gamma-amino butyric acid
Ig	immunoglobulin
LBO	lateral bulla osteotomy
MIC	minimum inhibitory concentration
MRI	magnetic resonance imaging
MRSA	methicillin-resistant *Staphylococcus aureus*
PCMX	parachlorometaxylenol
PVA	polyvinyl alcohol
TECA	total ear canal ablation
tris	tromethamine
VO	video-otoscope

1 THE NORMAL EAR

KEY POINTS

- The external ear comprises the pinna and the external acoustic meatus. It serves to collect and locate the origin of sound waves.
- The middle ear comprises the tympanic membrane, the ossicles, the auditory tube, and the tympanic cavity. It serves to transduce incoming airborne sound waves into waves in a liquid medium.
- The inner ear comprises the cochlea, the vestibule, and the semicircular canals. It interprets sound and serves to relate the head to gravity, allowing the visual system to compensate for movement and to perceive both linear and rotational acceleration.

INTRODUCTION

The ear of the dog and cat is composed of three parts: the external ear, the middle ear, and the inner ear (Figure 1.1)[1-3]. Together these components allow the animal to locate a sound and the direction from which it emanates, to orientate the head in relation to gravity, and to measure acceleration and rotation of the head. Selective breeding, of dogs in particular, has resulted in a wide variation in relative size and shape of the components of the external ear. Compare, for example, the French Bulldog, the Cocker Spaniel, the German Shepherd Dog, the St. Bernard, and the Persian cat. The pinnal shape and carriage, the diameter of the external ear canal, the degree of hair and amount of soft tissue within the external ear canal, and the shape of the

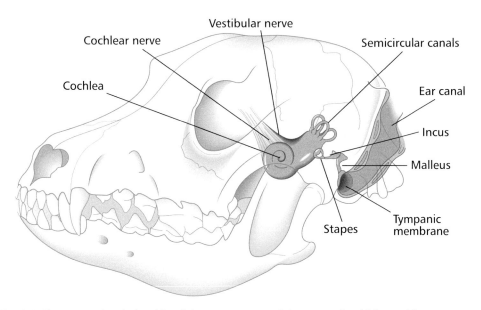

Fig. 1.1 The anatomic relationship of the components of the external, middle, and inner ear remains constant in relation to each other and the skull.

skull within which the middle and inner ear lie, vary from one breed to another. Despite this anatomic variation the essential relationship between the various components of the external, middle, and inner ear is preserved[1].

PINNA

The evolutionary role of the pinna has been as an aid to sound collection and point-of-origin location (Figures 1.2, 1.3). However, selective breeding of dogs has resulted in pinnae which often appear to have been designed more as lids to prevent access by foreign bodies (Figures 1.4, 1.5) or as vehicles to carry ornate displays of exuberant growths of hair (Figures 1.6, 1.7). Despite these changes, the functionality of the ear appears to have been maintained. In most breeds of cats the pinna is held erect, with the exception of the Scottish Fold Cat where the distal portion of the scapha is folded rostroventrally[4].

The pinna is composed of a sheet of cartilage covered on both sides by skin (Figures 1.2, 1.3), which is more firmly adherent on the concave aspect than on the convex aspect[2,3,5]. The cartilage sheet which supports the pinna is a flared extension of the auricular cartilage. Proximally this becomes rolled to form the vertical ear canal and part of the horizontal ear canal[6]. The major part of the external auditory meatus is contained within the auricular cartilage.

Generally the pinna is haired on the convex surface and in some breeds, such as the Cocker Spaniel and Papillon for example, markedly so. The concave aspect may be lightly haired on the free edges and towards the tip, but towards the base it becomes essentially glabrous and is tightly adherent to the underlying cartilage. A few fine hairs are usually present around the entrance to the external auditory meatus. In breeds with hirsute ear canals, such as Cocker Spaniels, there may be profuse hair growth along the whole length of the ear canal.

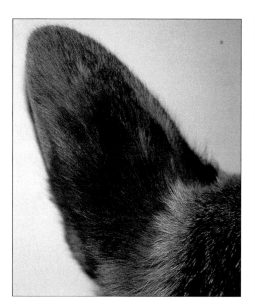 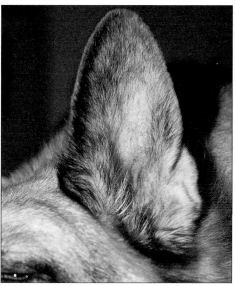

Figs. 1.2, 1.3 Archetypal pinna, in this case of a German Shepherd Dog. Note the even distribution of short hairs on the convex aspect (**1.2**). There is a variable amount of glabrous, sparsely-haired skin on the concave aspect (**1.3**) which is confluent with the epithelial lining of the external ear canal.

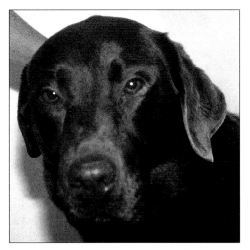
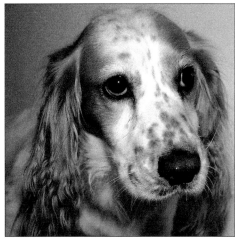

Figs. 1.4, 1.5 Examples of the various pinnae which have resulted from selective breeding. Labrador Retriever (**1.4**), Cocker Spaniel (**1.5**).

Figs. 1.6, 1.7 Examples of the various pinnae which have resulted from selective breeding. Papillon (**1.6**), Yorkshire Terrier (**1.7**).

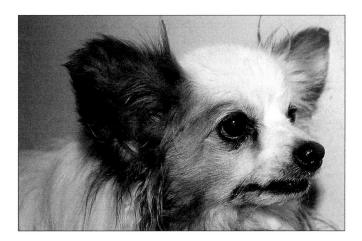

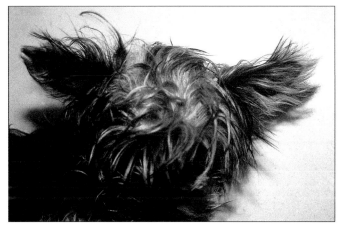

EXTERNAL AUDITORY MEATUS

The external auditory meatus serves to conduct sound waves to the tympanum. It is contained within the vertical and horizontal portions of the external ear canal. The size of the vertical canal (length and volume) correlates with body weight[7,8]. In the dog the average length of the external ear canal within the auricular cartilage is 4.1 cm (1.6 in) (2.2–5.7 cm [0.8–2.2 in]) and its average diameter, at the level of the tragus, is 5.8 cm (2.3 in) (2.1–7.9 cm [0.8–3.1 in])[7].

The vertical canal deviates medially, just dorsal to the level of the tympanum, towards the external acoustic process. In the dog the average length of canal within the annular cartilage is 1.2 cm (0.5 in) (0.8–1.9 cm [0.3–0.7 in])[7].

The epithelium and dermal tissues which line the bony and cartilaginous components of the external ear canal result in a smooth inner surface to the canal (Figure 1.8). The epithelium is sparsely haired in most, but not all, breeds, and it is rich in adnexal glands (see Microscopic structure of the external ear canal).

MIDDLE EAR

The middle ear and auditory (Eustachian) tube comprise a functional physiological unit with protective, drainage, and ventilatory capabilities[9,10]. The middle ear is composed of the tympanum, the ossicles, the auditory tube, and the tympanic cavities (Figure 1.9)[1,3]. The middle ear cavities are lined with secretory epithelium (Figure 1.10). Epithelia such as this not only secrete liquid, but also absorb gas[9]. This tends to result in a slight negative pressure within the normal middle ear cavity[9]. The composition of the gas in the normal middle ear cavity of both dogs and cats has been described[11]. It appears to correlate closely to the composition of the capillary blood, rather than reflecting gaseous exchange along the auditory tube.

The three ossicles transmit sound waves impacting upon the tympanic membrane to the oval window. At this point the mechanical energy of the ossicles is transduced to pressure waves within the inner ear, to be interpreted subsequently as sound. Pressure and internal homeostasis within the inner ear is equilibrated across the round window membrane.

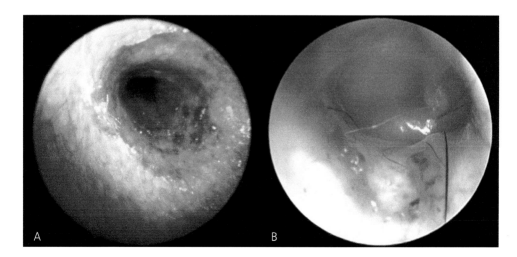

Fig. 1.8 Otoscopic picture of a normal canine (**A**) and feline (**B**) external ear canal, demonstrating the smooth epithelial lining. Note the occasional accumulations of cerumen.

Tympanum

The gross appearance of the canine and feline tympanic membrane is similar (Figure 1.8)[3,4,12]. The canine tympanum is a thin, semitransparent membrane with a rounded, elliptical outline; its mean size is 15–10 mm (0.6–0.4 in). The shorter dimension is nearly vertical, the long axis is directed ventral, medial, and cranial, and it has an area of approximately 63.3 mm² (0.1 sq in)[1,2,13]. The feline tympanum is more circular in shape (8.7–6 mm [0.3–0.2 in]) and has an area of approximately 41 mm² (0.6 sq in)[4,12,14]. The majority of the external

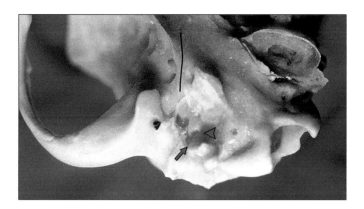

Fig. 1.9 The caudoventral aspect of a canine skull with the bulla removed. Three of the four ports of communication are visible: the external acoustic meatus (arrow), the round window on the promontory (arrow head), and the auditory tube (delineated with a piece of nylon).

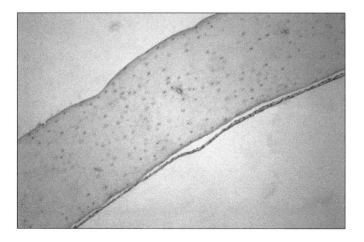

Fig. 1.10 Photomicrograph of a section of normal bulla. Note the thin bone and the secretory epithelial lining. (Sample prepared by Finn Pathology, Diss, Norfolk, UK.)

aspect of the tympanum is thin, tough, and glistening (the pars tensa) with the outline of the manubrium of the malleus being clearly visible (Figure 1.11). The manubrium inserts under the epithelium on the medial aspect of the tympanum and exerts tension onto it, resulting in a concave shape to the intact membrane, rather similar to the speaker cone in a loudspeaker[3,15]. The pars flaccida is more opaque, pink, or white in colour. It is confined to the upper quadrant of the tympanic membrane and bound ventrally by the lateral process of the malleus[3,13].

In a study of 100 cases of canine otitis externa, rupture of the tympanic membrane was negatively associated with underlying allergic disease and positively associated with grass awns, particularly in Cocker Spaniels[16].

MICROSCOPIC STRUCTURE OF THE EXTERNAL EAR CANAL

KEY POINTS

- The normal ear canal contains a stratified squamous epidermis, hair follicles, and associated sebaceous and ceruminous (apocrine) glands.
- Breeds of dog predisposed to otitis externa, such as Cocker Spaniels, have increased amounts of glandular tissue compared to other dogs.
- Otitis externa results in increased production of cerumen with a lower lipid content than normal, associated with increased ceruminous gland activity.
- Chronic otitis externa results in permanent changes.

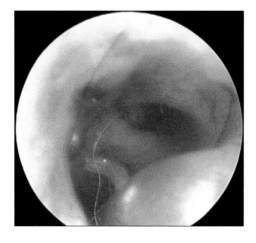

Fig. 1.11 Otoscopic picture of a normal tympanic membrane. The manubrium of the malleus is clearly visible.

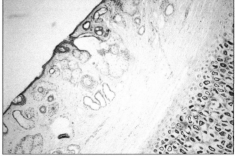

Fig. 1.12 Photomicrograph of a section of normal canine external ear canal illustrating the thin epidermis, which is only a few cells thick.

The epidermis lining the external ear canal is similar in structure to that of the interfollicular epidermis of the skin, i.e. a stratified cornifying epithelium with adnexal organs such as hair follicles and their associated sebaceous and ceruminous (apocrine) glands (Figures 1.12, 1.13)[1–4]. The underlying dermis is heavily invested with elastic and collagenous fibres (Figures 1.14, 1.15). Beneath the dermis and subcutis lie the rolled cartilaginous sheets of the auricular and annular cartilages which contain and support the external ear canal.

Hair follicles

All breeds of dog have hair follicles throughout the length of the external ear canal, although in most breeds these follicles are simple and sparsely distributed (Figure 1.16)[3]. It has been suggested that the density of hair follicles decreases as one progresses toward the external acoustic meatus[1,2], but recent studies[3,4] did not describe such a distribution. The mean proportion of integument occupied by hair follicles was found to be 1.5–3.6%, with no significant spatial distribution

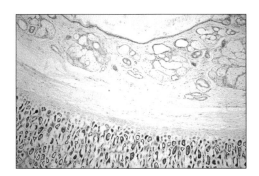

Fig. 1.13 Photomicrograph of a section of normal feline external ear canal. Note the thin epidermis, the sparse hair follicles, sebaceous glands, and ceruminous glands, and the underlying auricular cartilage.

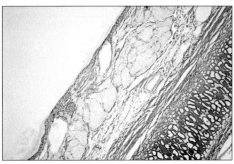

Fig. 1.14 Photomicrograph of a section of normal canine external ear canal stained with Gomorri's stain to highlight collagen and fibrous tissue in the dermis.

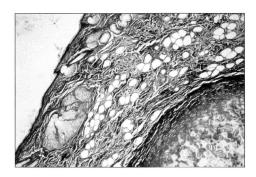

Fig. 1.15 Photomicrograph of a section of normal canine external ear canal stained with Masson's stain to highlight collagen and fibrous tissue in the dermis.

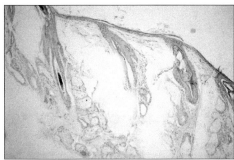

Fig. 1.16 Photomicrograph of a section of normal canine external ear canal showing simple hair follicles.

along the canal. There was a large interdog variation[4].

However, some breeds which are predisposed to otitis externa differ from the basic pattern[3]. Thus, Cocker Spaniels exhibit a much higher concentration of hair follicles than other breeds and, furthermore, the follicles are typically compound in pattern (Figure 1.17)[3]. There is no correlation between the percentage of hair follicles within the otic integument and predisposition to otitis externa[4].

Hair is sparse or absent in the feline external ear canal[5].

Adnexal glands

Sebaceous glands are present in the upper dermis[1–5,6]. They are numerous and prominent (Figure 1.18) and have a similar structure to the sebaceous glands of the skin. The mean proportion of integument occupied by sebaceous glands is 4.1–10.5%, gradually increasing from proximal to distal and peaking at the level of the anthelix[4]. There is a large interdog variation[4]. The sebaceous glands secrete principally neutral lipids[4]. In the normal dog this lipid accounts for the majority of the cerumen, along with sloughed

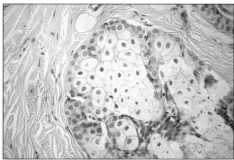

Fig. 1.18 Photomicrograph of a section of normal canine external ear canal showing a higher power view of a sebaceous gland.

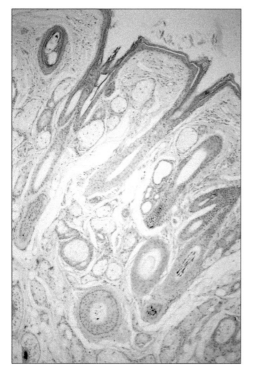

Fig. 1.17 Photomicrograph of a section of normal canine external ear canal from a Cocker Spaniel. Note the density of the hair follicles compared to **1.16** and that they are compound.

epidermal debris[7]. This high lipid content of normal cerumen helps maintain normal keratinization of the epidermis, aids in the capture and excretion of debris both produced within and entering the external ear canal, and results in a relatively low humidity within the lumen of the ear canal. In the cat the sebaceous glands become more prevalent and crowded proximally[5].

Ceruminous (apocrine) glands are located in the deeper dermis (Figure 1.19)[1-5]. They are characterized by a simple tubular pattern and a lumen lined by a simple cuboidal-pattern epithelium. In the normal dog and cat the ducts of the apocrine glands are virtually nonapparent. The mean proportion of integument occupied by apocrine glands is 1.4–4.5%, gradually decreasing from proximal to distal and peaking at the level of the tympanic membrane[4]. There is a large interdog variation[4]. The apocrine glands contain acid mucopolysaccharides and phospholipids[5].

Overall, these data[4] suggest that the ratio of apocrine to sebaceous gland decreases from proximal to distal, tending to produce a more aqueous cerumen in the deeper ear canal, possibly more conducive to epidermal migration. The more lipid nature of cerumen at the distal end may facilitate water repulsion.

MICROCLIMATE OF THE EXTERNAL EAR CANAL

KEY POINTS

- The principal factor affecting the microflora within the external ear canal is the microenvironment.
- Temperature and relative humidity within the external ear canal are very stable.
- The mean temperature within the external ear canal is between 38.2°C (100.7°F) and 38.4°C (101.1°F), some 0.6°C (33.1°F) lower than the rectal temperature.
- The mean relative humidity in the external ear canal is 88.5%.
- The mean pH of the normal external ear canal is 6.1 in males and 6.2 in females.
- Otitis externa is associated with a rise in relative humidity and a rise in pH within the external ear canal.
- Cerumen is composed principally of lipid and sloughed epithelial cells.
- In cases of chronic otitis externa, the lipid component of cerumen decreases.

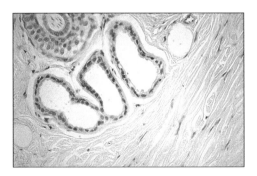

Fig. 1.19 Photomicrograph of a section of normal canine external ear canal showing a higher power view of an apocrine gland.

Epithelial lining

The external ear canals are lined such that the underlying cartilaginous architecture and the intercartilaginous joints are covered by a smooth, clean epithelial surface (Figure 1.20). The epithelial surface is composed of closely apposed squames which are covered by a variable, but usually thin, layer of cerumen and adherent debris (Figures 1.21, 1.22). There is a constant, outward movement of cerumen[1,2]. Squames detach (Figures 1.23, 1.24) and move distally in the cerumen, thus keeping the tympanum clear of debris and providing a mechanism for removing sloughed epithelial and glandular secretions from the external ear canal.

Temperature

In a series of studies the temperature within the external ear canal of dogs was 38.2–38.4°C (100.7–101.1°F)[3–5]. These studies were performed over a span of 25 years with very different technologies, and for such close results to be achieved is remarkable. There was no significant difference between breeds of dog or whether there was a pendulous pinna or not[3,4]. The temperature within the external ear canal rises significantly if otitis externa is present: mean 38.9°C (102°F)[5]. The temperature within the external ear canal is a mean of 0.6°C (33.1°F) lower than rectal temperature.

One study[3] was performed in Australia where the environmental temperature tends to be high. Nevertheless, as the day grew progressively hotter the temperature within the external ear canal only rose by 0.3°C (32.5°F) compared to a rise of 6.4°C (43.5°F) in the environment. This illustrates very well how the environment within the ear canal is effectively buffered from the external environment.

Relative humidity

In one study the mean relative humidity within the external ear canal of 19 dogs was 80.4%[6]. This was remarkably stable throughout the day[6], with a recorded rise within the ear of only 2.3% compared to 24% in the external environment, again illustrating the buffering effect of the tissues surrounding the external ear canal. Grono[6] suggested that the high relative humidity in the external ear canal was such that the meatal epithelium would readily become hydrated and macerated, an ideal environment for bacterial proliferation. In cases of otitis externa, the relative humidity was somewhat higher (mean 89%) than normal, but not significantly so. The influence of a pendulous pinna was not reported.

pH

The range of pH in normal dogs is between 4.6 and 7.2[6]. The mean pH is slightly lower in males than in females (6.1 compared to 6.2). The pH rises in otitis externa. Grono[7] measured the pH in cases of otitis externa and found the mean to be 5.9 (range 5.9–7.2) in acute cases and 6.8 (range 6.0–7.4) in chronic cases. Grono also measured the pH of the external ear canals of dogs and recorded the bacteria which

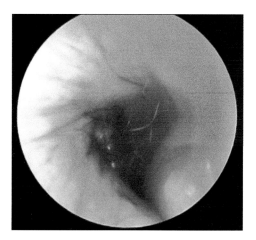

Fig. 1.20 Otoscopic view of the normal external ear canal. Note the clean, smooth epithelial surface.

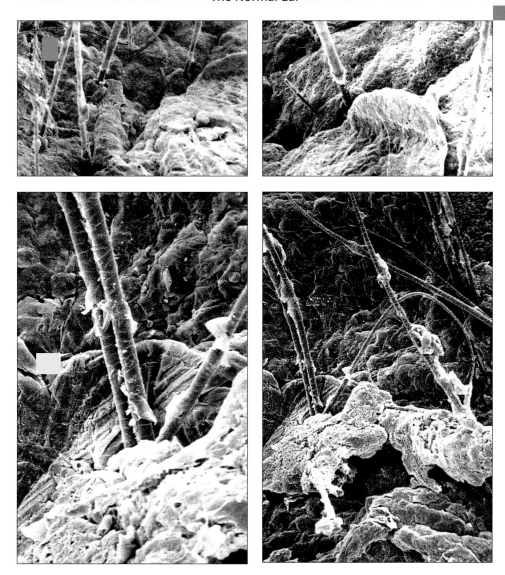

Figs. 1.21, 1.22 Scanning electron micrographs of the epithelial surface of the external ear canal of a dog (**1.21,** top) and a cat (**1.22,** above). Note the cerumen coating the hair shafts and squames such that individual squame borders cannot clearly be seen. (Electron micrographs produced by the Department of Anatomy, Royal Veterinary College, London, UK.)

Figs. 1.23, 1.24 Scanning electron micrographs illustrating squames in the process of detaching in a canine ear canal (**1.23,** top) and a feline ear canal (**1.24,** above). (Electron micrographs produced by the Department of Anatomy, Royal Veterinary College, London, UK.)

were isolated from some of these cases. Nonparametric (Mann Whitney) analysis of Grono's data by the authors showed that in cases of otitis externa associated with *Pseudomonas* spp., the pH is significantly higher (mean 6.85, $p<0.05$) than in cases of otitis externa in which no *Pseudomonas* spp. are isolated (mean 5.7).

CERUMEN IN NORMAL AND OTITIC EARS

Cerumen coats the lining of the external ear canal (Figures. 1.25, 1.26). It is composed of lipid secretions from the sebaceous glands, ceruminous gland secretion[8], and sloughed epithelial cells. The lipid component of dogs' cerumen can vary widely, as does the type of lipid within the cerumen, although margaric (17:0), stearic (18:0), oleic (18:1), and linoleic (18:2) fatty acids are the most common[9,10]. A range of 18.2–92.6% (by weight) of lipid content was found in the external ear canals of normal dogs, and in some cases there was wide disparity between the left and right ears. This variation presumably reflects individual variation in concentration and activity of ceruminous glands. In man, cerumen type ('wet' or 'dry') is a simple mendelian trait[11]. Whether there is a simple genetic control of canine or feline cerumen type is not known. Oleic and linoleic acid have antibacterial activity[12,13], although the effects of these fatty acids, and others, against bacteria and *Malassezia pachydermatis* within the ear canal is less clear[10].

In cases of otitis externa the lipid content of the cerumen falls significantly to a mean of 24.4%, compared to a mean of 49.7% from normal ears[9]. This fall in lipid content may reflect the hypertrophy of apocrine glands which accompanies chronic otitis externa[14]. The decreased lipid component of cerumen may account for the increase in relative humidity reported in the external ear canals of dogs with otitis externa[6]. This, plus the decrease in antibacterial activity, may allow increased bacterial multiplication.

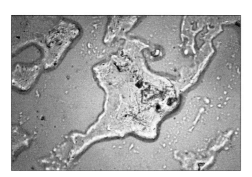

Fig. 1.25 Photomicrograph of normal cerumen. Note the high proportion of amorphous lipid material to squame.

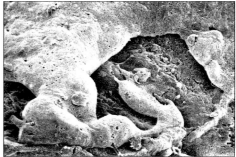

Fig. 1.26 Scanning electron micrograph illustrating cerumen on the epithelial surface of a cat's external ear canal. (Electron micrograph produced by the Department of Anatomy, Royal Veterinary College, London, UK.)

2 APPROACH TO THE DIAGNOSIS OF OTITIS EXTERNA

INTRODUCTION

The approach to a case of otitis externa is no different to that of any disease:

- A look at the signalment will allow the clinician to consider breed, age, and sex predisposition to otitis externa.
- A case history may be sufficient to allow a working diagnosis of a foreign body to be made.
- In other cases it may be apparent that the dog has suffered occasional bouts of bilateral otitis externa before and, in these cases, a more detailed approach is necessary.

Consideration of the history and signal–ment will allow the clinician to make a provisional differential diagnosis, which will be further amended once the physical examination has been performed. At this point, a number of investigatory techniques can be utilized to stage the otitis (*Table 2.1*).

Table 2.1 Investigative techniques that may be employed in order to stage otitis externa

Visual examination and palpation of the auricular cartilages

Otoscopic/video-otoscopic examination of the external ear canal

Cytological examination of cerumen and exudate

Sampling for culture and sensitivity testing of exudate

Cleaning the ear canal to facilitate examination of the deeper canal and tympanic membrane

Radiography, including canalography

Histopathological examination of biopsy samples

SIGNALMENT

Breed

Some breeds, for example Cocker Spaniels and Persian cats, are predisposed to defects in keratinization, which may be associated with a ceruminous otitis externa. Breeds of dog recognized as particularly prone to otitis externa include Springer Spaniels, Miniature Poodles, Shar Pei, and German Shepherd Dogs. Any breed predisposed to atopy is likely to exhibit (usually) bilateral otitis externa. Dogs with pendulous pinnae are not necessarily predisposed to otitis externa but they may be susceptible to a rapidly progressive infection, should otitis externa develop. Breeds with excessive hair within the external ear canals, such as Poodles, may be predisposed to accumulations of cerumen and debris, which may provoke otitis externa. Yorkshire Terriers are predisposed to bilateral pinnal alopecia and hyperpigmentation. Cocker Spaniels were predisposed to grass awn-related acute otitis externa in one study of 100 cases[1].

Longhaired breeds of cats and show cats are commonly affected by dermatophytosis. White haired cats and dogs are predisposed to actinic radiation damage to the pinnae.

Age

Young animals are often affected with *Otodectes cynotis*, but this may not be associated with pruritus, particularly in kittens. In cats, the peak incidence of otitis externa is between 1 and 2 years of age, presumably reflecting exposure to, and hypersensitivity to, *O. cynotis*. In older cats bilateral otitis externa is almost always associated with *O. cynotis* infection, whereas unilateral otitis externa may reflect cat bite abscess or obstructive otitis secondary to polyps or neoplasia. Young animals are predisposed to dermatophytosis.

In dogs, young animals (and very old animals) are under-represented in studies of the incidence of otitis externa. The peak incidence of otitis externa occurs in dogs between 3 and 6 years of age. Otic foreign bodies are unusual in young animals. Underlying disease, such as a defect in keratinization, atopy, or a dietary intolerance, may cause uni- or bilateral otitis externa and may occur in young animals, particularly in predisposed breeds.

Sex

There is no sex predisposition to otitis external in general, although one study found that females were more likely than males to exhibit allergic pattern otitis[1]. Sertoli cell tumour may be associated with a greasy cerumen which adheres to the skin and hair adjacent to the orifice of the external ear canal.

HISTORY

The key aims of history taking are:
- In some cases to allow a definitive diagnosis, thus allowing specific treatment.
- More usually, to identify whether or not there is any evidence of management or underlying disease which may be predisposing the animal to otitis externa.

The history should encompass all aspects of the dog's management and lifestyle in an attempt to identify the cause of the otitis externa.

Management and lifestyle
- Diet: to identify deficiencies such as zinc and essential fatty acids.
- Water intake: any polyuria/polydipsia?
- Housing: kenneled or indoors?
- Exposure to sunlight: actinic radiation damage.
- Exercise: swimming predisposes to ear disease.
- Work: (working dogs predisposed to foreign bodies).
- Grooming requirements: clipper burn on the pinnae, failure to pluck the ear canals, otic irritation following plucking, contagion at clipping parlour?
- Presence of other animals (*O. cynotis*, *Sarcoptes scabiei*, dermatophytosis).
- Hunting cat (*Spilopsyllus cuniculi*, feline poxvirus infection, ticks).

Evidence of underlying disease
- Recurrent episodes of ear disease should raise the suspicion of an underlying disease, particularly if bilateral.
- Facial, otic, and pedal pruritus suggest atopy.
- Erythema in the ear, facial, neck, and truncal folds, and perhaps crust, scale, and erythema on the pinnae and trunk, suggest a defect in keratinization.
- A seasonal pattern is most likely to reflect atopy or seasonal exposure to ectoparasites such as mosquitoes, flies, harvest mites (*Neotrombicula* spp.), and rabbit fleas (*S. cuniculi*).
- Dietary intolerance is often associated with otitis externa.
- Allergic contact dermatitis may affect the concave, ventral aspect of the pinnae.

- Endocrinopathies may be associated with a ceruminous otitis externa.
- Sudden onset of severe, ulcerative bilateral otitis, perhaps in association with other skin disease, or systemic signs should raise the suspicion of drug eruption or immune-mediated disease.

Medications
Topical application of otic medication may induce an irritant or allergic contact dermatitis. The clinical sign which might suggest this is continued otitis in the face of repeated application of a medication. Neomycin is the most often cited agent in this regard, although propylene glycol also may be irritant.

PHYSICAL EXAMINATION

Having established the immediate and past history, the dog should be given a full clinical examination. In particular, evidence of internal disease and endocrinopathies should be sought. Thus, lymph nodes and testes should be palpated, the oral cavity examined, the chest auscultated, the abdomen palpated, and the perineum checked. Only after this general physical examination should the dermatological assessment take place.

Pinnal scratch reflex
In some pruritic canine dermatoses, rubbing the distal edge of the pinna between finger and thumb nail induces a scratch reflex from the ipsilateral hindlimb. This positive scratch reflex is most commonly associated with scabies, although it is not pathognomonic. Pediculosis, *Malassezia pachydermatis* dermatitis, and atopy also may result in a positive scratch reflex.

OTIC EXAMINATION

Gross examination of the pinnae

- Peripheral crust and scale may suggest scabies, pediculosis, a defect in keratinization, zinc deficiency, endocrinopathy, or fly bite or mosquito hypersensitivity.
- Erythema on the convex aspect, particularly distal, suggests actinic radiation damage.
- Erythema on the concave aspect suggests atopy or allergic contact dermatitis.
- Alopecia may be due to pruritus (scabies, pediculosis, hypersensitivity) or dermatophytosis.
- Alopecia and hyperpigmentation may reflect an endocrinopathy.
- Curling of the pinnae in the cat is almost pathognomonic for relapsing polychondritis.
- Vesicles, pustules, and crust may be due to superficial pyoderma, pemphigus foliaceus, or zinc deficiency.
- Punched out ulcerations on the convex aspect may be due to feline cowpox.
- Punched out ulcerations on the concave aspect and pinnal margin may reflect vasculitis.

Gross examination of the external ear canal

- Calcification of the otic cartilage, which can be palpated, suggests the presence of chronic otitis externa.
- Malodour of the external ear canal may be associated with *M. pachydermatis* infection, gram-negative bacterial infection, devitalized tissues, or neoplasia.
- The amount of hair around the entrance to and within the external ear canal should be assessed. The clinician may need to remove this hair in order to complete an auroscopic examination.
- The areas hidden within the cartilage folds at the entrance to the ear canal should be examined for ectoparasites, particularly ticks and trombiculid mites.
- Erythema is often associated with swelling of the soft tissues of the external ear canal and stenosis of the lumen. In some cases the stenosis is so severe that it is impossible to insert the cone of an otoscope into the canal. Erythema of the vertical canal, in combination with a normal, or nearly normal, horizontal canal is very suggestive of atopy.
- Ulceration of the otic epithelium is usually associated with gram-negative bacterial infection but it may be a sign of immune-mediated disease.
- The nature, colour, and odour of any discharge should be noted. However, whether any conclusions as to the causal organism, based on the physical nature of the discharge, are valid is debatable. Cytological examination of the discharge is much more reliable in this regard.

OTOSCOPIC APPEARANCE OF THE EXTERNAL EAR CANAL AND TYMPANUM

KEY POINTS

- Do not examine the ear in isolation. Obtain a history and examine the animal first.
- Ear canals may require cleaning before a proper examination is possible.
- Always examine both ears, even if a unilateral problem is suspected.
- Adequate restraint is essential; use of a sedative or neuroleptanalgesia is often required. Be prepared to administer general anaesthesia, if necessary.
- Cats require general anaesthesia before they are subjected to otoscopic examination.
- Remember that the presence of hair in the external ear canal is normal in some dogs.
- Do not expect to visualize *O. cynotis* unfailingly: otic cerumen mixed with liquid paraffin and examined under a microscope will allow a better chance of diagnosis if mite numbers are low.

Sedation for otoscopy and aural examination

In order to examine the entire length of the ear canal properly, adequate restraint is necessary as the external ear canal must be manipulated into as straight a line as possible. This is achieved by gently grasping the pinna and pulling it, and the attached auricular cartilage, up and away from the sagittal plane.

Otoscopic cannulae are hard, often cold, and have sharp ends. It hurts when a cannula is thrust into an inflamed ear canal. Although video-otoscopes have a narrow probe, the same constraints apply. In most cases, and particularly with small dogs and cats and animals with painful or tender ear canals, this process is resented and the animal will require chemical restraint or general anaesthesia.

McKeever and Richardson[1] advocate a mixture which provides approximately 20 minutes of sedation, sufficient to allow thorough examination and cleaning of both ears:

- Ketamine (1.36–2.2 mg/kg).
- Midazolam (0.023 mg/kg).
- Acepromazine (0.023 mg/kg).
- All mixed in the same syringe and injected slowly iv.

An alternative would be xylazine injection (1–2 mg/10 kg i/v), which should provide about 20 minutes of reasonable sedation.

Another alternative is detomidine (20–40 µg/kg i/v), which will produce moderate sedation and has the great advantage that it can be reversed by intramuscular injection of its antagonist atipamezole. Note that there are two disadvantages with this regime: it is very expensive (mitigated by giving buprenorphine at the same time), and there is a risk of inducing a cardiac arrhythmia if potentiated sulphonamides are administered at the same time.

Normal appearance of the external ear canal and tympanum

The normal external ear canal is smooth, pale in colour, and contains minimal discharge (Figures 2.1, 2.2). A small amount of pale yellow or brown cerumen (Figures 2.3, 2.4) may be seen in some cases and this is normal[2]. Occasionally, there may be a hair shaft in the horizontal canal (Figures 2.5, 2.6). In some breeds, such as Cocker Spaniels, Miniature and Giant Schnauzers, Airedales, and other terriers, for example, there are hair follicles the

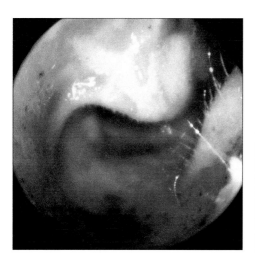

Fig. 2.1 The upper portion of the feline external ear canal.

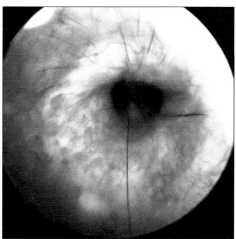

Fig. 2.2 A normal horizontal external ear canal of a dog. There is an even, pale colour with a smooth contour. A few fine hairs may be seen.

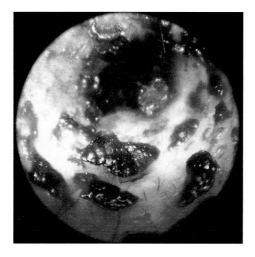

Fig. 2.3 Patchy brown cerumen adhering to the walls of a normal external ear canal.

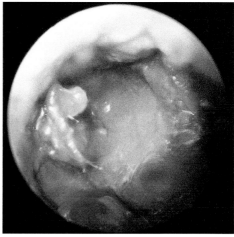

Fig. 2.4 Yellowish cerumen near the tympanum.

whole length of the external ear canal[1-3]. The diameter of the vertical portion of the external canal varies from breed to breed but at its base, where it apposes the horizontal portion, it is 5–10 mm (0.2–0.4 in) in diameter[3]. The horizontal canal is approximately 2 cm (0.8 in) in length[3].

The normal tympanum is thin, pale grey in colour (described as rice paper-like), and translucent (Figure 2.7). It is visible via otoscopy in about 75% of normal ears[4]. Cerumen, debris, or hair prevents a clear view of the tympanum in the other ears[4]. The shape of the tympanum is

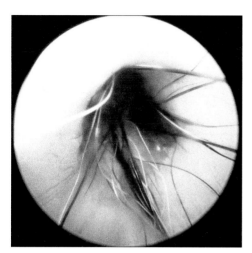

Fig. 2.5 Tufts of hair emerging from the horizontal ear canal.

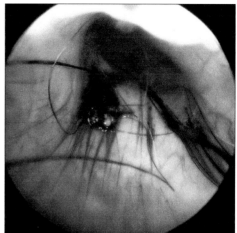

Fig. 2.6 Hair and adhering cerumen emerging from the horizontal ear canal.

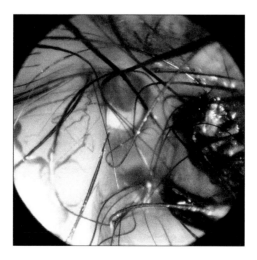

Fig. 2.7 A normal, translucent tympanic membrane, in this instance partially hidden by hair and cerumen.

elliptical, mean 15×10 mm (0.6×0.4 in), with the short axis nearly vertical[2]. The initial otoscopic view is restricted to the posterior quadrant of the pars tensa and the pars flaccida[5, 6]. Manipulation of both the external ear canal and the otoscope will usually bring the majority of the manubrium (Figure 2.8) and the larger portion of the pars tensa into view[5,6]. The external aspect of the tympanum, as viewed with an otoscope, is divided into two unequal parts by the manubrium of the malleus. This is attached along the medial aspect of the tympanum and exerts tension onto it, resulting in a concave shape to the intact membrane.

Abnormal appearance of the external ear canal

Inflammation results in oedema, erythema, and warmth (Figure 2.9). Given that the glandular tissues of the external ear canal are contained within a cartilaginous tube, any swelling will result in a reduction in the diameter of the lumen. In many cases the concave aspect of the pinna will also be affected (Figure 2.10). In most cases the inflammation affects the entire ear canal, but in some instances it will be localized to either the horizontal or, more usually, the vertical canal. Bilateral inflammation confined to the concave aspect of the pinna and the vertical canal, particularly if there is little discharge, is very suggestive of atopy (Figure 2.11). Indeed, erythema of the entire canal in the absence of significant discharge or other pathology is highly suggestive of allergy. Atopy, dietary intolerance, and neomycin sensitivity should all be considered in the differential diagnosis.

Inflammation also results in increased secretion from the glands within the epithelial lining of the canal and a shift away from a lipid to an aqueous constitution[7,8]. Continued inflammation results in maceration of the stratum corneum, loss of barrier function, and the outward movement of transepidermal fluid. Discharge accumulates within the external ear canal (Figures 2.12–2.14) and microbial proliferation

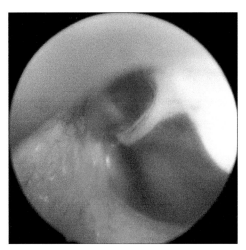

Fig. 2.8 The tympanic membrane with the manubrium of the malleus clearly visible.

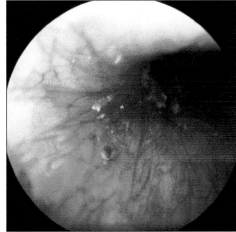

Fig. 2.9 Erythematous otitis in a case of atopy. There is erythema and some degree of swelling, resulting in loss of luminal cross-section.

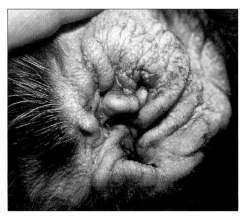

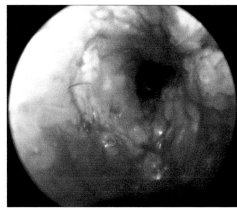

Fig. 2.10 External ear canal of an atopic dog. There is erythema, hyperplasia, and lichenification.

Fig. 2.11 Erythema, hyperplasia, moderate fissure formation, and a tendency to ulcerate and bleed very easily, even after otoscopy, are commonly seen in ear canals of atopic dogs.

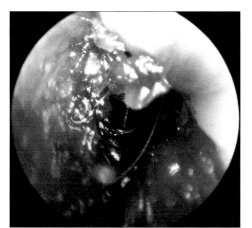

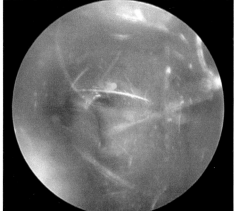

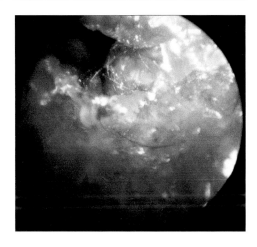

Figs. 2.12–2.14 Three views showing erythema, hyperplasia, cerumen, and varying degrees of luminal stenosis.

occurs. The colour of the discharge may vary from light yellow to dark brown and it may be aqueous, thin, or pus-like in nature. Animals with severe or generalized defects in keratinization may exhibit a greasy yellow discharge that has a purulent appearance, but which may be free of pathogens and noninflammatory in nature. Medications may result in a thin, shiny covering over the mural epithelium.

The presence of erosions and ulcers in the external ear canal should be noted (Figure 2.15). Frank ulceration is uncommon and is usually associated with gram-negative bacterial infection. Rare causes of otic ulceration are autoimmune diseases and otic neoplasms. The finding of ulcers within the external ear canal mandates samples for both cytological evaluation and bacterial culture and sensitivity testing.

Otoscopic examination may reveal the presence of ectoparasites, such as *O. cynotis* or *Otobius megnini* (Figure 2.16). Otodectic mites are often accompanied by the presence of a crumbly brown discharge (Figure 2.17). Not all infestations are inflammatory. Failure to detect otodectic mites during otoscopic examination does not preclude infestation, and microscopic examination of cytological samples is necessary.

Epidermal hyperplasia, nodules, tumours, polyps, and foreign bodies within the external ear canal are easily visualized during otoscopy (Figure 2.18), although cleaning of the external ear canal may be necessary. This is particularly the case for cats where the whole canal may fill with purulent discharge if an otic tumour or polyp is present (Figure 2.19).

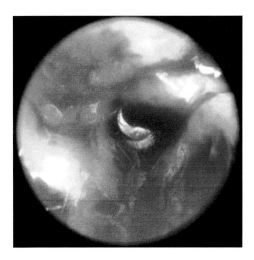

Fig. 2.15 Haemorrhagic foci associated with focal ulcerations in a case of gram-negative infection.

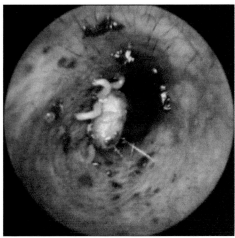

Fig. 2.16 Spinous ear tick, *Otobious megnini*, within the vertical ear canal. (Courtesy of Dr. Louis Gotthelf, DVM; Montgomery, AL, USA.)

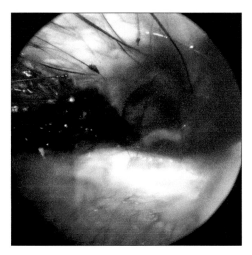

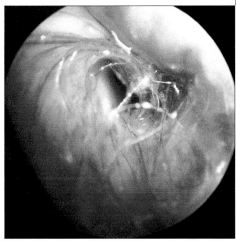

Fig. 2.17 Crumbly, dry, blackish brown cerumen associated with *Otodectes cynotis* infestation.

Fig. 2.18 Grass awn, cerumen, and associated erythema in the external ear canal of a dog.

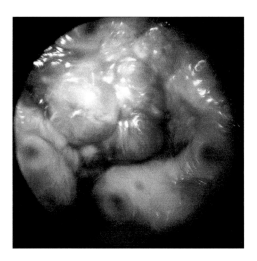

Fig. 2.19 Polyp in the external ear canal of a cat.

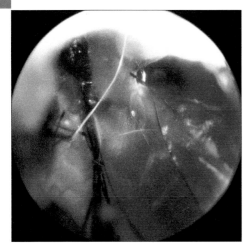

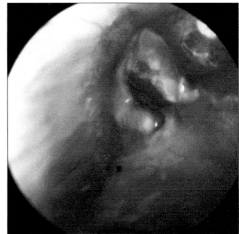

Fig. 2.20 Acute tear in the tympanic membrane of a dog associated with grass awn penetration.

Fig. 2.21 Chronic otitis media and otitis externa have resulted in a thickened, opaque, ruptured tympanic membrane.

The tympanum should be examined for colour, texture, and integrity; it is usually dark grey or brown in cases of otitis externa[1]. In contrast to normal dogs, it is only possible to visualize the tympanum adequately in 28% of ears affected with otitis externa[4]. If tears or holes in the tympanum (Figures 2.20, 2.21) indicate that otitis media is present (although an intact tympanum does not rule out otitis media), then failure to visualize the tympanum adequately, let alone a tear, suggests that diagnosis of otitis media, exclusively via otoscopy, is not reliable. Bulging of the tympanum may indicate an accumulation of exudate within the middle ear, whereas retraction (and a concave appearance) suggests a partially filled middle ear with obstruction of the auditory tube[5].

Tympanic defects may heal in the presence of infection in the middle ear. Thus, diagnosing otitis media on the sole basis of a ruptured tympanum is unreliable.

CYTOLOGICAL CHARACTERISTICS OF NORMAL AND ABNORMAL EARS

- Cytological samples should be taken before ear cleaning is undertaken.
- Both external ear canals should be sampled, preferably from the horizontal canal.
- There is no reliable correlation between the physical nature of the discharge and a particular microbe.
- Examination of unstained, oil-mixed cerumen is a reliable method of determining infestation with *O. cynotis*.
- Information on the organisms within the canal and the type and nature of the inflammatory response may be obtained from microscopic examination of stained smears; modified Wright's stains, such as Diff-Quik, are ideal stains for in-house use.

Introduction

Otodectic otitis (Figure 2.22) is often associated with a crumbly, rather dryish discharge (Figure 2.23), similar to coffee grounds[1]. However, there is no clear-cut relationship between the gross characteristics of any otic discharge and the species of micro-organism with which it is associated, e.g. staphylococcal, gram-negative, or malassezial[2,3].

Cytological examination of otic exudate is a rapid, in-house test which provides diagnostically and therapeutically useful information[2–5]. Reproducibility is high with regard to detecting micro-organisms and is good for bacteria, but is less so for yeast[6]. In many cases, information from cytological examination of cerumen is more accurate than that from samples submitted for microbiological culture and sensitivity testing. Furthermore, the clinician can assess the significance of any micro-organisms in the light of other ceruminal characteristics, such as the presence of nucleated squames, proteinaceous debris, and inflammatory cells. This is particularly exemplified in the case illustrated (Figure 2.24) of a Cocker Spaniel with

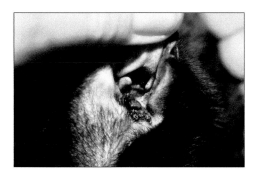

Fig. 2.22 Typical appearance of cerumen associated with *Otodectes cynotis* – dark, dry, and crumbly. As in this case, it is not always associated with inflammation in the ear canal.

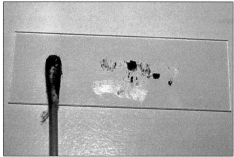

Fig. 2.23 The dry, crumbly nature of the cerumen can be appreciated when it is rolled onto a glass slide.

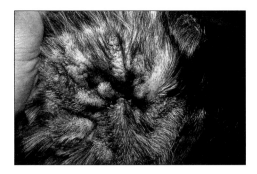

Fig. 2.24 External ear canal of a Cocker Spaniel with chronic otitis externa.

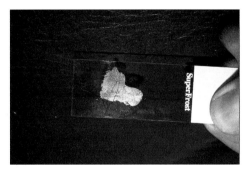

Fig. 2.25 Gross appearance of an unstained cytologic sample – thick and white.

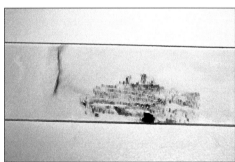

Fig. 2.26 Gross appearance of a Diff-Quik-stained sample – thick and blue, suggestive of a high cell content.

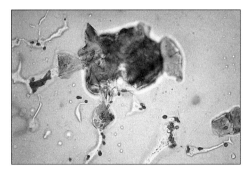

Fig. 2.27 High-power photomicrograph from the Cocker Spaniel in Fig. **2.24**. Note the yeast and cocci on and around the squames, and the absence of inflammatory cells.

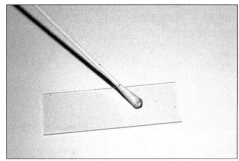

Fig. 2.28 Unstained smears from normal ear canals are all but invisible.

chronic, bilateral otitis associated with a thick, greasy exudate. Gross examination of the discharge (Figures 2.25, 2.26) might suggest that a malassezial, or even a gram-negative, infection was responsible but cytological examination (Figure 2.27) does not support this. Although there are increased numbers of squames and microbes visible, the lack of any inflammatory cells suggests a ceruminous otitis externa, probably associated with a more generalized defect in keratinization, rather than infection.

Samples and stains

The most useful sample for otic cytology is a swab taken from the ear canal, which is then rolled onto a clean glass slide. If feasible, samples should be taken from the horizontal portion of the external ear canal of both ears[4,5]. In large dogs it is usually possible to collect a shielded sample using, for example, an alcohol-sprayed otoscope cone. In small dogs and cats collecting a shielded sample is difficult, and vertical canal samples will have to suffice[5]. If otitis media is suspected, a shielded sample should be taken from the middle ear in addition to that from the external ear canal.

Most clinicians advocate using modified Wright's stains such as Diff-Quik[1,4,5]. Alcohol-based stains are more useful than aqueous preparations (e.g. new methylene blue) because of the lipid nature of the otic discharge[4]. Griffin[1] advocated heat fixing of obviously waxy preparations in order to prevent solvent-associated leaching of lipid. Since all cerumen contains lipid it would seem appropriate to heat fix all samples, but opinion is divided on this issue[4–8]. Subtle information may be lost if heat fixing is not performed, but generally it is not necessary unless samples are to be kept for future examination. Commercial laboratories usually perform a Gram's stain because, although more time consuming, it does allow assessment of the classification of organisms by both morphology (coccus, rod, diphtheroid) and Gram's stain status. Generally, Gram staining is too cumbersome and time consuming for practitioners to consider for a rapid, in-house stain[8].

Knowledge of morphology and Gram's stain status allows a recommendation for treatment[1,4]. In addition to allowing visualization of the microbial populations of the external ear canal, cytology also allows the physical nature of the cerumen to be assessed, in terms of keratinaceous debris and the lipid content of the cerumen[9,10].

Stained samples should be air-dried and examined for evenness of stain and for depth of stain, which is usually deeper in intensity as the cell count increases. A coverslip should be applied prior to microscopic examination[5]. Initial low-power examination is followed by high-power examination, and this is usually sufficient for accurate classification of any microorganisms and identification of any cells present[7,8].

Gross examination of cytological preparations

Gross examination of fresh and stained smears reflects the lipid and cellular content of cerumen. Normal cerumen has a high lipid content and a low concentration of intact cells, usually squames. Unstained preparations are all but invisible in direct light (Figure 2.28), reflecting the low cell content of cerumen. Increasing cell content, particularly if it is inflammatory in nature, is reflected in the increased opacity of the cerumen.

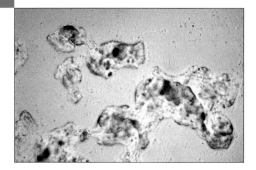

Fig. 2.29 Photomicrograph of a cytological sample from a normal ear. Note the low cell content in the cerumen.

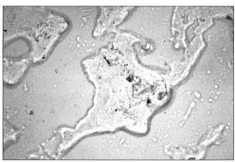

Fig. 2.30 Outlines of lipid are visible, even after fixing and staining with Diff-Quik.

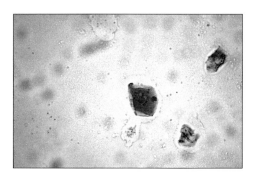

Fig. 2.31 Photomicrograph of a cytological sample from a normal ear, with a few squames apparent.

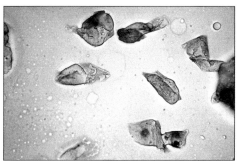

Fig. 2.32 Photomicrograph demonstrating increased numbers of squames, some of which are nucleated.

Normal cytological characteristics

Cerumen does not take up stain because of its high lipid content (Figure 2.29), although ghost outlines of lipid droplets may be seen occasionally (Figure 2.30). Low numbers of anucleate, epithelial cells may be detected, although in normal ears they are not excessive (Figure 2.31). When there is inflammation of the epithelial lining of the external ear canal, the rate of cellular turnover increases and nucleated squames may be seen in the cerumen (Figure 2.32). Low numbers of *Malassezia pachydermatis* and staphylococci may

be identified adhering to shed squames (Figures 2.33, 2.34). Leucocytes are usually absent from normal cerumen[4].

Abnormal cytological characteristics
Cerumen

The lipid content of cerumen from inflamed external ear canals is lower and the cell count is usually higher than that in normal ear canals[9]. This is reflected in the gross appearance of the stained smear, which appears bluer in a sample from an otitic ear (Figure 2.35) than in that from a normal ear (Figure 2.36).

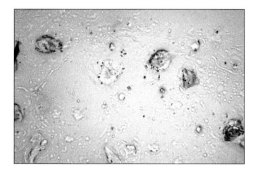

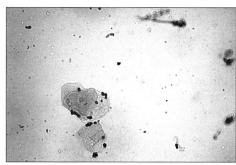

Fig. 2.33 Photomicrograph demonstrating a few anucleate squames with a few staphylococci apparent.

Fig. 2.34 Photomicrograph demonstrating a few anucleate squames with low numbers of yeast apparent.

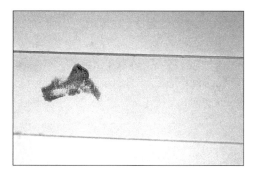

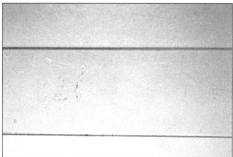

Figs. 2.35, 2.36 Gross cytological samples from an otitic and a normal ear canal. The otitic ear (**2.35**) contains a higher cell content and appears much bluer, when stained, than the smear from the normal ear (**2.36**).

Fig. 2.37 Photomicrograph from a case of otitis externa. There are anucleate and nucleated squames present.

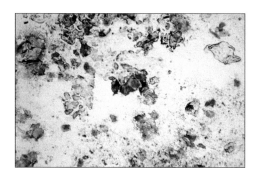

Keratinocytes

In acute cases of otitis externa, or cases of very short duration, there will be very little change in the epithelial shedding of squames. In chronic cases, such as those associated with defects in keratinization or atopy, the epithelial lining of the external ear canal reacts to the inflammation and the hyperplasia may result in the appearance of both anucleate and nucleated squames and debris (Figure 2.37).

Autoimmune disorders, in particular pemphigus foliaceus, may result in acantholysis. Single, nucleated, well-defined acanthocytes may be shed from erosions in the ear canal, often surrounded by adherent neutrophils (Figure 2.38), i.e. a positive Tzank test.

Inflammatory cells

In samples taken from dogs and cats with acute otitis externa there may be little change in the cellular population, but in most cases there will be neutrophils and proteinaceous debris (Figure 2.39). More chronic otitis results in the appearance of macrophages as well as neutrophils within the exudate[5]. In cases of bacterial otitis, the increasing concentration of toxins may result in the appearance of toxic neutrophils (Figure 2.40) and indicates that the external ear canal should be flushed before treatment is initiated[1].

Neoplastic cells

Intraluminal neoplasms may shed cells into the cerumen but it is unusual to find diagnostically useful material in this dis-charge[9]. Cells from adenocarcinomas tend to exfoliate in sheets or clusters, whereas squamous cell carcinomas shed large, densely-staining individual cells with prominent nucleoli (Figure 2.41)[5].

Bacteria

The normal microbial population of the ear canal is dominated by staphylococci. In the early stages of otic inflammation, the numbers of staphylococci increase, particularly the numbers of *Staphylococcus pseudintermedius* (Figure 2.42).

Care should be taken when pronouncing that staphylococci are present in cerumen or on the squames, as cocci may be confused with:

- Debris in poorly-maintained Diff-Quik (filter the stain regularly).
- Pigment granules within the squames (melanin granules are usually brown in colour rather than the blue-black colour of staphylococci).

Occasionally the otic flora remains staphy-lococcal in nature but most com–monly it becomes dominated by gram-negative

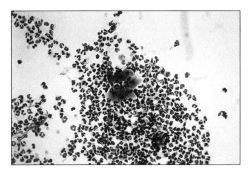

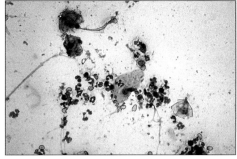

Fig. 2.38 Photomicrograph of a stained smear from a pustule in a case of pemphigus foliaceus. Compare the 'clean' neutrophils and rounded-up, nucleated squames in this Tzank test-positive smear with the cells and neutrophils in Figs. **2.39** and **2.40**.

Fig. 2.39 Photomicrograph of a small group of squames with surrounding neutrophils.

bacilli, in particular *Escherichia coli, Proteus* spp., and *Pseudomonas* spp. These changes in bacterial shape (i.e. coccoid to rod) are easily detected by microscopic examination of cytological samples (Figure 2.43)[5,7]. Cocci cannot be reliably classified as either staphylococci or streptococci on the basis of clumping or chain formation, respectively, since this is not usually observed[4]. With experience, clinicians may be able to detect that staphylococci are larger than streptococci[4].

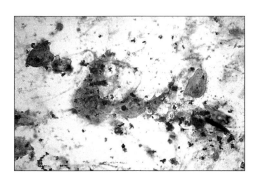

Fig. 2.40 Photomicrograph illustrating squames, proteinaceous debris, and dark, pyknotic neutrophils.

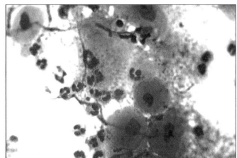

Fig. 2.41 Photomicrograph of cytological sample from an ear canal in which a squamous cell carcinoma was found. Note the typical appearance of the cells: large, densely staining with nucleoli.

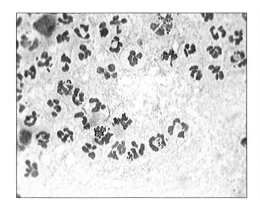

Fig. 2.42 Photomicrograph of a dense group of cells with large numbers of staphylococci apparent.

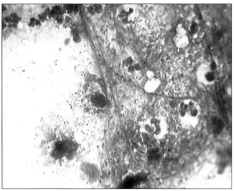

Fig. 2.43 Photomicrograph illustrating squames and vast numbers of bacilli.

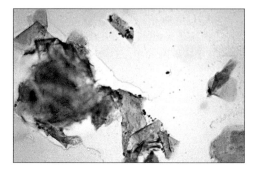

Fig. 2.44 Photomicrograph illustrating yeast.

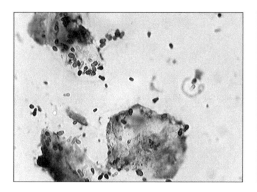

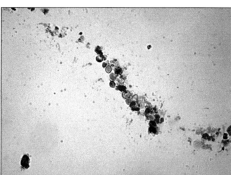

Fig. 2.45 Photomicrograph illustrating yeast in sufficient numbers to be associated with disease.

Fig. 2.46 Photomicrograph illustrating yeast and inflammatory cells.

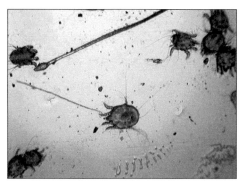

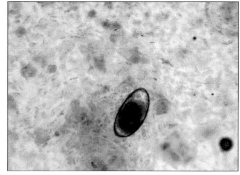

Figs. 2.47, 2.48 Photomicrograph of adult otodectic mites and an ovum recovered from the cerumen of an ear infected with *Otodectes cynotis*.

Generally, even in first opinion cases, the observation of bacilli should prompt sampling for bacterial culture and sensitivity testing[4]. This is particularly important if Gram staining is not performed, since clinicians cannot differentiate *Pseudomonas* spp. from *Clostridium* spp., or *Bacillus* spp.[4]. Unless a recurrent case is involved it is not usually necessary to submit samples from otitis externa associated with cocci for bacterial culture and sensitivity testing. Indeed, in one study, testing achieved a sensitivity of 59% for gram-positive cocci and 69% for gram-negative rods, compared with 100% sensitivity with cytological examination[8].

Yeast

M. pachydermatis is a member of the normal canine otic microflora[11], although it has the potential for opportunistic pathogenicity. At least two species of malassezial yeast can be isolated from feline ear canals, *M. pachydermatis* and *M. sympodialis*[12]. The presence of yeast (Figure 2.44) must, therefore, be interpreted with caution. Evidence of increased numbers of yeast (arbitrarily more than 5–10 per high-power field [Figure 2.45][1,4,5]) and an associated inflammatory reaction (Figure 2.46) should be sought before disease status is decided. Malassezial yeast are flask- or peanut-shaped, whereas candidial yeast are round in appearance, although this distinction is not easily made.

The importance of cytological evaluation was exemplified in two studies which reported that demonstration of malassezial infection by culture methods achieved a sensitivity of 82% and 50% respectively[1,8]. However, in another study looking at the reproducibility of cytology, the agreement for yeast organisms was only moderate[6]. In addition to relative insensitivity, malassezial culture is expensive and time consuming, resulting in unnecessary cost and delay in treatment compared to cytological assessment[2].

Ectoparasites

It is often easy to visualize *O. cynotis* and *O. megnini* within the external ear canal simply by using an otoscope. However, since very low numbers of mites have been associated with otitis externa[13] it is not surprising that they will be missed in some cases, particularly if there is an accumulation of debris or discharge within the canal. Therefore, microscopic examination of cytological preparations is indicated if otodectic mange is suspected. Cerumen is deposited on a glass slide and mixed with mineral oil prior to microscopic examination[2]. Otodectic mites have a characteristic appearance (Figures 2.47, 2.48).

Bacterial culture and sensitivity testing

In most cases, examination of cytological samples will provide all the information necessary for effective treatment to be instituted. Microbial culture and sensitivity testing of samples from the external ear canal is, however, useful in certain cases:
- In cases of recurrent, or refractory, otitis externa.
- If ulceration of the epithelial lining of the external ear canal is present.
- If gram-negative infection is suspected.
- If otitis media is suspected (when samples from the middle ear will also be necessary).

BIOPSY

Taking 4 mm (0.2 in) punch biopsy samples, under general anaesthesia, of the vertical ear canal or of lesions and masses within the external ear canal is an important method of obtaining useful information on the processes underway. Biopsy of the external ear canal has three main indications:

- As a means of providing information on the degree of permanence of epithelial changes. For example, some apparently permanently thickened epithelia will regress dramatically when treated with topical glucocorticoids to suppress the inflammatory reaction. However, fibrosis, in general, will not regress. Biopsy of the luminal wall can yield information on the degree of fibrosis present (see Chapter 1: Microscopic structure of the external ear canal). This information can help decide whether to opt for a surgical or medical approach.
- As a means of providing information on the aetiology of ulcerated lesions in the ear canal. Ulcers of the luminal wall may reflect gram-negative bacterial infection particularly, but also autoimmune disease and neoplasia. Biopsy of these lesions can yield information which will influence management.
- As an adjunct to surgery. Neoplastic changes within the ear canal may be fibrogranulomatous, benign, or malignant. Knowing the type of neoplasm and being able to predict its behaviour can help the surgeon plan the degree of resection necessary to remove the risk of recurrence.

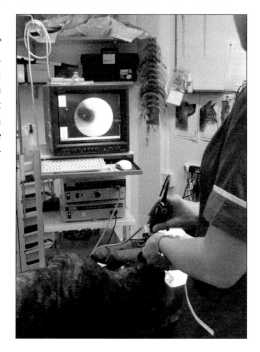

Fig. 2.49 Video-otoscope in a consulting room.

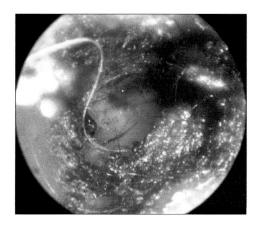

Fig. 2.50 Illustration of the quality of the image that can be obtained using a video-otoscope.

IMAGING

Video-otoscopic examination of the ear canal

The video-otoscope (VO) is a useful and effective tool in the management of both canine and feline otitis. Its widespread use is, unfortunately, limited by expense and it is most commonly available in referral institutions. The equipment takes up space in the consulting room (Figure 2.49). Although it has major advantages over hand-held otoscopes, animals do need to be minimally sedated but more commonly anaesthetized in order for it to be used successfully. Its uses and indications in veterinary medicine have been reviewed by different authors[1-3]. It has many advantages over the hand-held otoscope:

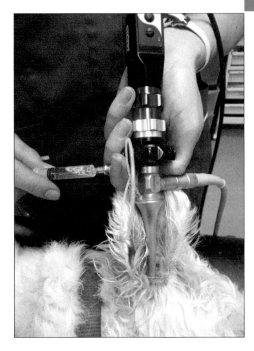

Fig. 2.51 In-use picture showing the workinghead inserted in a dog's ear canal.

- The VO provides a range of magnification lenses which allows assessment of fine detail especially at the level of the tympanic membrane (Figure 2.50). Often the inferior magnification of the hand-held instruments does not allow the clinician to see small tears in the tympanic membrane, which can be important when deciding on topical therapy.
- The intense light source which is positioned at the tip of the endoscope, rather than at the base of the cone as is the case with hand-held devices, provides excellent illumination to allow more detailed evaluation of the structures within the ear (Figure 2.51). This also prevents the problem of shadows within the visual field created when instruments are introduced down the working channels.
- The working channels facilitate fully visualized flushing (Figure 2.52) of the canal and removal of foreign bodies, such as grass awns or ceruminoliths, using grasping forceps.

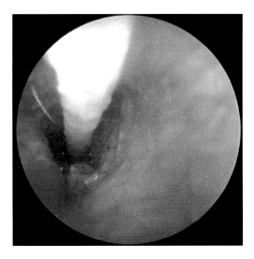

Fig. 2.52 Suction head within the external ear canal of a dog.

- Minor surgical interventions can also be performed. Biopsies may be taken from the canal using grasping forceps.
- Injections can be placed into the canal using a long hollow needle inserted down the working channel or by a rigid spinal needle inserted down alongside the otoscope cone.
- When samples are to be taken from the middle ear, in the face of an intact tympanic membrane, myringotomy can be performed safely, because important structures to be avoided, such as the malleus and pars flaccida, can be visualized.
- Some VOs, especially those with wide working channels, can also be used with lasers which can be used to ablate small lesions in the walls of the canal or to perform myringotomy.
- Modern VOs allow photographic documentation of clinical cases which helps enhance the patient's medical record and can be used to provide colleagues and the client with a pictorial record; often the ability of an owner to see the ear canal of their pet, especially when comparisons are made with a normal ear, leads to increased owner compliance with therapy.

Virtual otoscopy for evaluating the inner ear

The technique of virtual otoscopy depends on manipulating computed tomography (CT) data with commercial software[1,2]. Although beautiful images are generated, the technique has little practical application at present.

Radiography

Radiographic examination is a useful tool in the investigation of ear disease in both the dog and the cat. Principally, it is utilized for the diagnosis of disease affecting the middle ear, although there are some indications for radiographic examination of the external ear canal.

KEY POINTS

- Careful positioning is the key to radiographic interpretation of the tympanic bullae.
- The most useful views are the dorsoventral, rostrocaudal (open mouth), and lateral oblique views.
- Given the individual variation between animals, comparison of one side with the other is often the only way of making a diagnosis. Therefore, perfect positioning is essential.

The radiological anatomy of the petrous temporal bones, and the associated components of the middle ear, is complex and subject both to breed and individual variation, particularly in the dog[1-5]. Consequently, a thorough knowledge of the spatial relationships between the skull and the ear is essential if the radiographs are to be interpreted correctly[3]. However, pathological changes to the region are unlikely to be symmetrical. Thus, provided a good quality, symmetrical radiographic image is obtained, useful information may be acquired by comparing one side with the other[2,3].

Normal radiographic features

- Dolichocephalic (or oligocephalic) heads are long and narrow, e.g. as in the Rough Collie and Saluki.
- Mesaticephalic heads are more rounded, e.g. as in the Doberman Pinscher and Labrador Retriever.
- Brachycephalic heads are short and wide, e.g. as in the English Bulldog and the Pekingese.

Any one of several radiographic views will provide information on the middle ear but no one view can provide a complete picture. Therefore, at least two different radiograph views must be included in any radiographic investigation. The three most frequently used radiographic views are the lateral oblique, the dorsoventral, and the rostrocaudal (open mouth) views. Lateral and ventrodorsal views may occasionally be required.

Lateral oblique view (Figures 2.53, 2.54)

Advantages: Good visualization of the tympanic bulla and petrous temporal bone.

Disadvantages: General anaesthesia is necessary. Only one bulla can be visualized at a time. Not easily repeatable, even in the same animal, so side-to-side comparison is difficult[6].

Positioning: The animal is placed in lateral recumbency with the head parallel to the film and the bulla of interest nearest the film. The jaw should be closed. Either the head is rotated around this long axis until the sagittal plane lies at about 20° to the horizontal, the bulla to be radiographed remaining ventral, or the nose is elevated some 15–20% to achieve separation of the bullae on the plate[6]. The beam should be centred to the base of the ear to project the bulla clear of other structures.

Interpretation: The bullae appear as thin-walled, crisply outlined bone structures with a smooth external border (Figures 2.55, 2.56)[7]. Air shadow

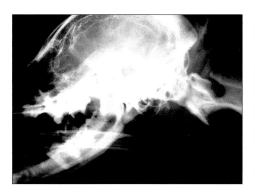
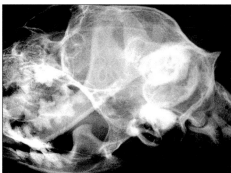

Figs. 2.53, 2.54 Lateral oblique radiographs of the head of a dog (**2.53**) and a cat (**2.54**) demonstrating optimal positioning for visualizing the tympanic bullae, which are clearly visible.

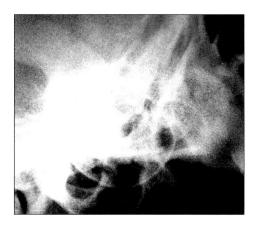
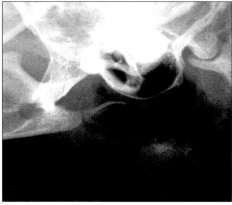

Figs. 2.55, 2.56 Close-up view of the normal tympanic bullae of a dog (**2.55**) and a cat (**2.56**) in the lateral oblique view.

should be visible in the external ear canal[7]. Predominantly lytic changes on the rostroventral wall of the bulla are usually associated with chronic inflammation[7]. Lytic changes within the petrous temporal bone may reflect either inflammation or neoplasia[7,8].

Rostrocaudal (open mouth) view
(Figures 2.57, 2.58)

Advantages: Good visualization of both tympanic bullae. Good view for diagnosing otitis media[4,9].

Disadvantages: General anaesthesia is necessary and the endotracheal tube must be removed. Can be difficult to obtain perfect pictures without fine-tuning, especially with brachycephalic breeds.

Positioning: The animal must be in dorsal recumbency. The head is positioned with the sagittal plane and hard palate vertical to the film. The tongue must be brought as far forward as possible and tied to the mandible with tape[8]. The interpupillary line must be parallel to the film. In dolichocephalic breeds the primary beam is centred through the open mouth parallel to the hard palate[5]. In mesaticephalic breeds it may be necessary to angle the hard palate slightly away from the vertical (perhaps 10° or so[4]). In brachycephalic breeds the hard palate may need to be angled up to 20° away from the vertical in order to avoid superimposing the bullae on the wings of the atlas[5]. Alternatively, the centre of the beam can be angled rostrocaudally, at up to 30° angling towards the hard palate. The beam can be centred on the base of the tongue[10].

Interpretation: The bullae appear as thin-walled, symmetrical bone opacities at the base of the skull (Figure 2.59)[7]. Overlying soft tissues may produce the appearance of middle ear pathology. This must be interpreted with care.

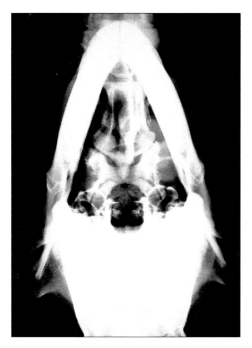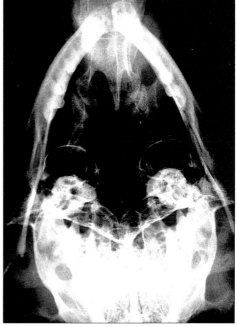

Figs. 2.57, 2.58 Rostrocaudal (open mouth) radiographs of the head of a dog (**2.57**) and a cat (**2.58**) demonstrating how the tympanic bullae are skylined.

Optimizing the diagnosis of otitis media by imaging

Several studies have tried to ascertain whether radiography, ultrasound, or CT alone, or in combination, are optimal for visualizing disease in the canine and feline bulla[11–13]. In summary:

- Few clinicians have access to CT.
- No technique is definitively better than any other in detecting both the presence and severity of middle ear disease.
- Ultrasound is a very useful modality, particularly in the case of investigating the feline bulla.
- Given that many veterinary practices have access to both ultrasound and radiography, the combination of both will give added diagnostic confidence.

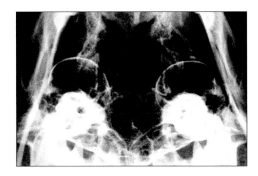

Fig. 2.59 Close-up rostrocaudal (open mouth) view of the tympanic bullae of a cat. Near perfect positioning is important for this view as one is looking for subtle changes that may only be apparent by comparing one side with the other.

Dorsoventral view (Figures 2.60, 2.61)

Advantages: Anaesthesia may not be necessary, although in most cases it will allow better positioning. In some patients sedation may suffice. It is easier to achieve good bilateral symmetry with this view than with the ventrodorsal

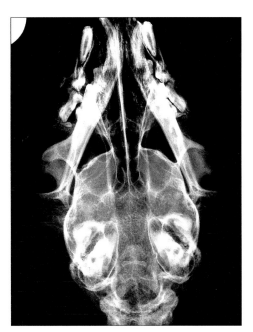

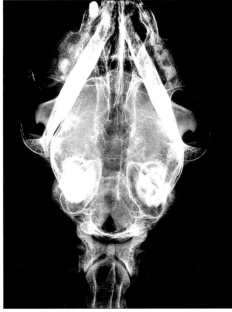

Figs. 2.60, 2.61 Dorsoventral radiographs of the head of a dog (**2.60**) and a cat (**2.61**). Note the appearance of the bullae and the difficulty in visualizing them using this position compared with the lateral oblique and rostrocaudal (open mouth) views.

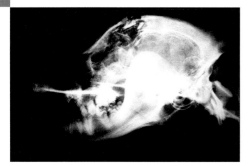 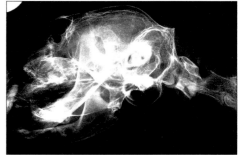

Figs. 2.62, 2.63 Lateral radiographs of the head of a dog (**2.62**) and a cat (**2.63**). The bullae are visible but both left and right bullae are superimposed, making interpretation difficult.

view, as the mandibles provide stability against lateral rotation[6]. Provides a good view for diagnosing otitis media[4].

Disadvantages: Because the calvarium is further from the plate it is magnified and this can induce some artefactual distortion[6]. However, this is more than outweighed by the advantage of having the bullae close to the plate.

Positioning: The animal is placed in ventral recumbency, under general anaesthesia or heavy sedation. Care must be taken to ensure that the animal is aligned symmetrically with the inter-pupillary line parallel to the film[6]. The hard palate must be parallel to the table and the animal adjusted so that the base of the skull is as close to the film as possible[6]. This may require support with radiolucent blocks of foam under the rostral mandible, sandbags over the cervical spine, or both. The beam should be centred at the intersection of two imaginary lines: a sagittal line, and a lateral line, at right angles to the sagittal line, drawn through the estimated position of the tympanic membranes.

Interpretation: The bullae should exhibit bilateral symmetry and appear as fine, crisp, distinct, linear bony opacities[7].

Some distortion and masking may occur due to superimposition of the petrous temporal bones[6]. Air shadow should be visible in the external ear canals.

Lateral view (Figures 2.62, 2.63)

Advantages: Standard view; lots of reference material.

Disadvantages: General anaesthesia is necessary. Not ideal for visualizing individual tympanic bullae as they are superimposed if a true lateral position is achieved.

Positioning: The animal is placed in lateral recumbency and the head adjusted to true lateral, with the sagittal plane parallel to the film and the interpupillary line vertical[6]. This may require foam padding to achieve a true lateral. The calvarium, nasal pharynx, and larynx should be included in the view. The beam should be centred between the ear and the eye.

Interpretation: The bullae appear as thin-walled, crisply outlined bony structures with a smooth external border (Figures 2.64, 2.65), but in a true lateral view they will be superimposed, making for difficult interpretation[6]. Air shadow and, if present, the thickened walls of the horizontal ear canal, may be visible[6].

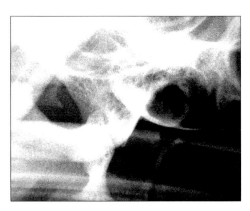
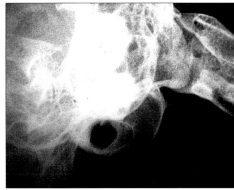

Figs. 2.64, 2.65 Close-up views of the tympanic bullae of a dog (**2.64**) and a cat (**2.65**) demonstrating the air shadow of the horizontal ear canal.

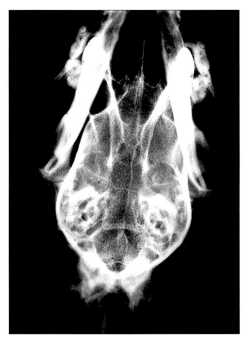
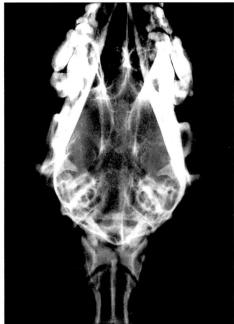

Figs. 2.66, 2.67 Ventrodorsal radiographs of a dog (**2.66**) and a cat (**2.67**). Note the appearance of the bullae and the difficulty in visualizing them using this position compared with the lateral oblique and rostrocaudal (open mouth) views.

Ventrodorsal view (Figures 2.66, 2.67)

Advantages: Standard view; lots of reference material. Provides a good view for diagnosing otitis media[4].

Disadvantages: Requires general anaesthesia. This position is not suitable for brachycephalic breeds[5]. The sagittal crest tends to make the skull fall laterally, making exact positioning difficult[6].

Positioning: The animal is placed in dorsal recumbency, under general anaesthesia. Care must be taken to ensure that the animal is aligned symmetrically. The hard palate must be parallel to the table. This may require support under the rostral mandible or under the cervical spine, or both. Intraoral tape, positioned immediately caudal to the canine teeth and then tied to the table, may help in positioning the mandible. The beam should be centred at the intersection of two imaginary lines: a sagittal line, and a lateral line, at right angles to the sagittal line, drawn through the estimated position of the tympanic membranes.

Interpretation: The superimposition of the petrous temporal bones makes the bullae walls appear thicker, and this can make evaluation of subtle changes more difficult. The bulla of the cat contains an additional inner bony wall which appears in this view (Figure 2.67)[6].

Visualizing the external ear canal and assessing the tympanic membrane

Radiography is not commonly employed as a means of assessing pathological changes in the external ear canal. It may be possible to see air shadows (Figures 2.68, 2.69) delineating the external ear canal in some of the standard radiographic views of the ear, particularly the dorsoventral and rostrocaudal (open mouth) views. In addition, in cases of chronic otitis externa, there may be calcification of the cartilages of the external canal (Figures 2.70–2.72). However, it is not possible to assess the integrity of the tympanic membrane or visualize the position of an obstructing luminal neoplasm without using contrast techniques.

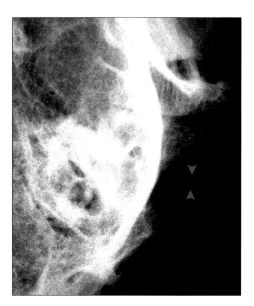

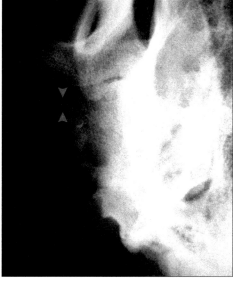

Fig. 2.68 Dorsoventral radiograph of a Cairn Terrier with a normal ear. The air shadow within the external ear canal is visible (arrowheads).

Fig. 2.69 Dorsoventral radiograph of a West Highland White Terrier with chronic otitis externa. In this close-up of the right side of the skull, the narrow ear canal is visible between the thickened walls of the horizontal ear canal (arrowheads).

Otoscopic and plain radiographic examinations must be performed prior to contrast studies. Significant epidermal hyperplasia or neoplastic proliferation may occlude the lumen to such an extent that adequate distribution of contrast medium is impossible. In addition, the presence of an exudate or mass within the bulla may prevent contrast medium from entering the middle ear. False-negative interpretation may occur if these changes are not identified prior to contrast studies[14].

A standard radiographic contrast medium is used, preferably a nonionic, water-soluble iodine-based medium rather than an oily medium[14]. The contrast medium may be diluted 50:50 with saline prior to instilling it into the

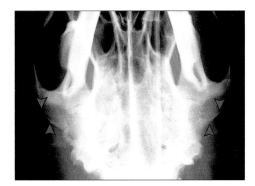

Fig. 2.70 Dorsoventral radiograph of an Airedale Terrier showing early signs of calcification of the external ear canal cartilages (arrowheads).

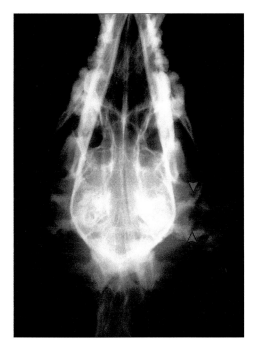
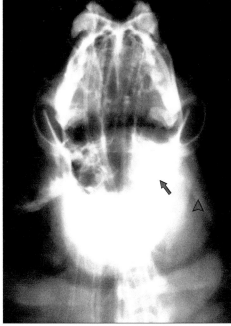

Figs. 2.71, 2.72 Dorsoventral and rostrocaudal (open mouth) radiographs of a Cocker Spaniel with chronic otitis externa and otitis media. Note the extensive calcification of the ear canal cartilages (arrowheads) and the changes around the left bulla (arrow).

external ear canal[14]. Care must be taken to ensure that the contrast medium is distributed evenly along the external ear canal and that none contaminates the hair on the surrounding aspects of the head[3,14]. Gentle massage of the ear canal will ensure an even distribution. Taking care to deliver all the contrast medium into the ear canal, and subsequently plugging the orifice with cotton wool, should prevent soiling of the area around the external ear[3,14].

Ventrodorsal or, preferably, rostrocaudal (open mouth) radiography will allow evaluation of the lumen of the external ear canal and permit some deductions on the state of the tympanic membrane (Figure 2.73)[15]. If contrast medium enters the middle ear (Figure 2.74) it is usually visualized as an opacification of the inner wall of the bulla[11], best seen on rostrocaudal (open mouth) views. Failure to detect contrast medium in the bulla should not be interpreted as indicating an intact tympanum.

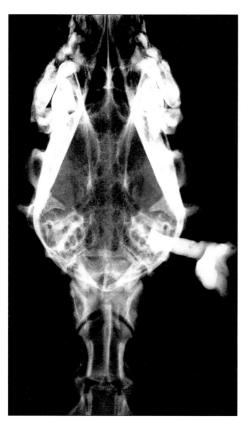 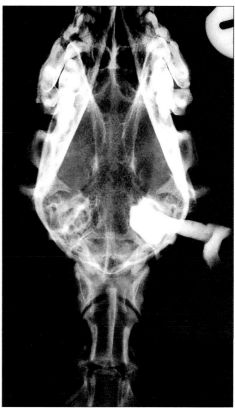

Figs. 2.73, 2.74 Ventrodorsal radiographs demonstrating tympanography. In Fig. **2.73** the tympanum is intact and the concavity is apparent. In Fig. **2.74** the tympanum has been breached and contrast fills the tympanic bulla.

3 AETIOLOGY AND PATHOGENESIS OF OTITIS EXTERNA

CONCEPT OF PRIMARY AND SECONDARY FACTORS, PREDISPOSING FACTORS, AND PERPETUATING CHANGE

August[1] proposed that the approach to otitis externa should not be considered symptomatically, but through the identification and management of three factors. He proposed a triad of primary, predisposing, and perpetuating factors. Although this system provided a basis for investigation and treatment of ear disease for many years it has more recently been superseded by the PSPP System[2]:

- Primary (P) and Secondary (S) causes are diseases or infectious agents that directly cause inflammation in the ear.
- Perpetuating (P) and Predisposing (P) factors are agents or elements that contribute to ear disease. Factors do not cause ear disease in their own right but can prevent resolution of disease and can lead to recurrence.
- Both causes and factors contribute to ear disease and both need to be identified and addressed to resolve disease.

This concept helps form the basis of a logical approach to otitis externa and each case should be considered in the following, non-exclusive classification:

- Is there a primary cause? Primary causes are capable of causing otitis externa in their own right and include allergy, autoimmune disease, endocrine disease, ectoparasites, epithelialization disorders, foreign bodies, glandular disorders, immune-mediated disease, micro-organisms, and viral disease (*Table 3.1*).
- Are there secondary causes present? Secondary causes normally contribute to or cause pathology in an abnormal ear. Secondary causes are the easiest to identify and in the early stages of the disease the easiest to treat. However, where they become chronic or recurrent it is usually because a primary cause or a perpetuating factor has not been adequately addressed. It is important not to focus entirely on the secondary cause of otitis at the expense of the primary cause. The most important secondary causes are bacterial and yeast infection, the use of inappropriate medication, or over cleaning (*Table 3.2*).
- Are there perpetuating factors? Perpetuating factors are changes in the anatomy and physiology of the ear that occur as a consequence of otitis externa. They tend to aggravate the otitis and further induce pathological changes within the lining of the external ear canal. Perpetuating factors include changes to the ear

canal epithelium, tympanum, and glandular structures in the wall of the canal as well as otitis media, which may occur as a consequence of otitis externa (*Table 3.3*) and is commonly underdiagnosed in chronic cases of otitis externa. Perpetuating factors may initially be mild but as the disease process progresses they often become the most significant part of the ear disease, and accentuate secondary causes due to chronic damage creating an environment within the ear to enhance bacterial and yeast growth.

Table 3.1 **Primary causes of otitis externa**

	Types
Allergy	Adverse food reaction, atopic otitis, contact allergy
Autoimmune	Bullous pemphigoid, epidermolysis bullosa, lupus erythematosus, pemphigus foliaceous
Ectoparasites	*Otodectes cynotis, Otobius megnini, Demodex* spp., *Eutrombicula* spp.
Endocrine	Hyperadrenocorticism, hypothyroidism, Sertoli cell tumour, sex hormone abnormalities
Epithelialization disorders	Primary idiopathic seborrhoea, sebaceous adenitis, zinc responsive dermatosis, vitamin A responsive dermatosis, idiopathic inflammatory otitis of the Cocker Spaniel
Foreign bodies	Hair, grass awns, sand, dirt
Glandular disorders	Hypersecretory states, sebaceous gland abnormalities
Immune mediated	Erythema multiforme, vasculitis, drug eruption
Micro-organisms (rare)	Fungi (*Aspergillus* spp.)
Miscellaneous	Eosinophilic granuloma complex, juvenile cellulitis, proliferative perforating otitis of kittens
Viral	Canine distemper

Table 3.2 **Secondary causes of otitis externa**

	Types
Bacteria	Cocci (staphylococcus, streptococcus, enterococcus)
	Baccilli (*Pseudomonas* spp., *Proteus* spp., *Escherichia coli, Klebsiella* spp., *Corynebacteria* spp.)
Yeast	*Malassezia* spp., *Candida* spp.
Medication reaction	Products containing topical irritants (alcohol, low pH, propylene glycol)
Over-cleaning	Water-based solutions causing maceration (water, water-based cleaners, antibiotics in aqueous solution); dry cleaning with cotton wool

- Are there any predisposing factors? Predisposing factors (*Table 3.4*) make otitis externa more likely by changing the internal environment in such a fashion that humidity within the ear canal rises, surface maceration occurs, and microbial proliferation follows.
- Predisposing factors include:
  - Conformational factors such as the amount of soft tissue within the confines of the auricular cartilage.
  - The presence of hair follicles, particularly compound hair follicles, within the external ear canal.
  - Stenotic ear canals (Shar Pei) or hair within the ear canal (Cocker Spaniel).
  - Water within the external ear canal either through swimming or from grooming may precipitate acute gram-negative infection or *Malassezia pachydermatis* otitis externa.
  - The external environment may also be pertinent since humidity and high temperature are known to be correlated with an increased incidence of ear disease.

Although predisposing factors will not cause ear disease they can, on occasion, combine with secondary causes and engender otitis externa. For example, obstructive ear disease caused by neoplastic or hyperplastic lesions can lead to changes in the environment in the ear, predisposing to infection and subsequent disease.

Table 3.3 Perpetuating factors for otitis externa

	Types
Ongoing pathological changes within the ear canal	Failure of epithelial migration, oedema, proliferative change, canal stenosis, calcification of pericartilagenous fibrous tissue
Tympanum	Acanthosis, dilation, rupture, diverticulum or pocket
Glandular tissue	Apocrine blockage and dilation, hidradenitis, glandular hyperplasia
Middle ear (otitis media)	Material within the middle ear (granulation tissue, infection, foreign material, primary secretory otitis media)

Table 3.4 Predisposing factors for otitis externa

	Types
Conformation	Hairy ear canals, pendulous pinna, stenotic ear canals, hairy concave pinna
Excessive moisture	Environment (heat and high humidity), water (swimmer's ear, grooming)
Obstructive ear disease	Neoplasia, polyps, cyst
Systemic disease	Debilitation, immunosuppression
Treatment effects	Trauma from cleaning, over-use of antibiotics

PRIMARY CAUSES OF OTITIS EXTERNA

Hypersensitivity

KEY POINTS

- Atopy is the most common cause of chronic canine otitis; it is a rare cause of feline ear disease.
- Otitis associated with dietary intolerance appears to be more severe that that seen in atopy.
- Irritant contact dermatitis of the external ear canal may be due to exposure to one of the common vehicles in otic preparations (e.g. propylene glycol) or to an active ingredient (e.g. neomycin).

Atopy is an inherited predisposition to develop immunoglobulin (Ig) E to environmental allergens resulting in disease[1]. Affected dogs exhibit pruritus and otitis externa[1-3]. Atopy has been stated to be the most common cause of chronic otitis externa in dogs[3]. The incidence of otitis externa in atopic dogs has been estimated at 55% and in 3% of atopic dogs otitis externa was the only clinical sign[2]. Atopy does exist in cats and will cause otitis externa in this species, although rarely.

Otitis externa in atopic dogs often begins as erythema at the base of the concave aspects of the pinnae and on the vertical portions of the external ear canals (Figures 3.1, 3.2)[1]. The horizontal portion of the external ear canal is minimally affected in early cases. Scott[2] reported that otitis externa associated with atopy often flared in association with the skin disease. This is a valuable clue that an alert clinician should spot when taking a history.

Atopy is associated with erythema and oedema of the ear canal but there is usually little exudation[2]. Secondary changes and microbial proliferation result in extension of these early clinical signs to the horizontal canal and hyperplasia of the epithelial lining (Figure 3.3). Malassezial proliferation may be particularly troublesome (Figure 3.4). Although chronic otitis externa is commonly due to atopy, it rarely results in gram-negative bacterial infection.

Lateral wall resection or vertical canal ablation should not be carried out on an atopic ear in an attempt to alleviate the otitis externa, without an appreciation of the underlying disease. The inflammation will continue to affect the medial and lateral walls of the residual canal and the proximal aspect of the pinna (Figures 3.5, 3.6).

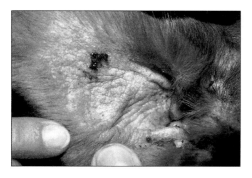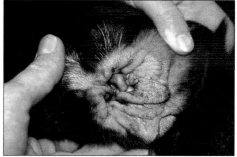

Figs. 3.1, 3.2 Classic signs of a hypersensitivity affecting the proximal aspect of the concave side of the pinna (3.1) and the upper portions of the external ear canal (3.2). There is erythema and hyperplasia in both areas.

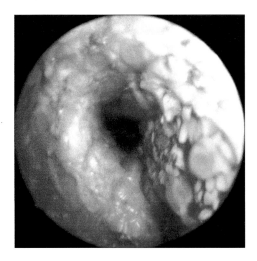

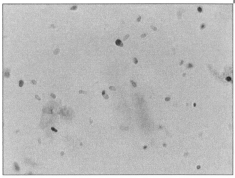

Fig. 3.4 Photomicrograph of a cytological sample taken from an atopic dog's external ear canal. There are a few squames, no inflammatory cells, but many yeast.

Fig. 3.3 Otoscopic picture of the lower portion of the vertical ear canal of a dog with atopy. Note the erythema and hyperplasia.

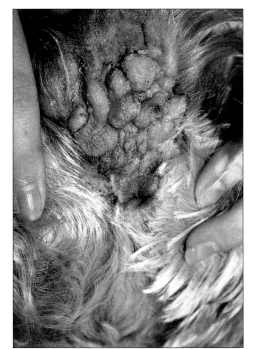

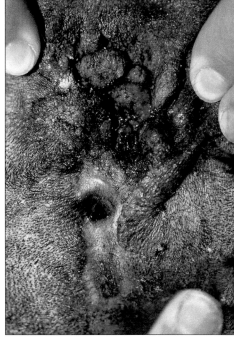

Fig. 3.5 Failed lateral wall resection in an atopic West Highland White Terrier. Persistent erythema and hyperplasia continue to affect the residual medial wall of the external ear canal.

Fig. 3.6 Only partially successful vertical canal ablation in an atopic dog. Erythema and hyperplasia still affect the proximal aspect of the pinna and the residual portion of the medial wall of the external ear canal.

Dietary intolerance

Dietary intolerance is a dermatosis which is much less common than atopy. However, when it occurs there may be concurrent otitis externa. Although otitis externa may, on rare occasions[4], be the only sign of dietary intolerance, it is commonly associated with other signs, typically pruritus[4-6]. The otitis associated with dietary intolerance appears to be more severe that that seen in atopy and it exhibits a rapid progression. Otitis externa is also associated with dietary intolerance in cats[6,7].

Contact dermatitis

Allergic contact dermatitis is a rare dermatosis in dogs and is almost unknown in cats[8]. In dogs with very extensive or generalized allergic contact dermatitis, the concave aspects of the pinnae and upper portion of the vertical ear canals may exhibit lesions (Figure 3.7)[9].

More commonly, allergic contact dermatitis or irritant contact dermatitis may occur due to exposure to any of the components of an otic preparation, provided it is used for long enough. Irritant contact dermatitis within the confines of the external ear canal may be due to exposure to one of the common vehicles, propylene glycol[10].

However, the most commonly implicated component is neomycin, although documented, published reports are very rare. Bilateral, erythematous otitis externa would be anticipated (Figure 3.8). The classic history is a cat or dog with chronic, relapsing otitis externa, which had previously responded well to a certain medication only to deteriorate when exposed to the medicant again.

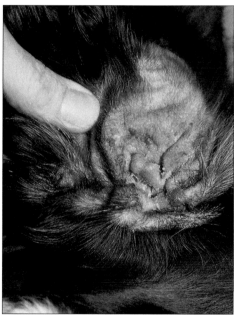

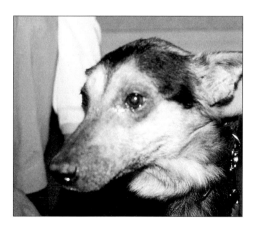

Fig. 3.7 Allergic contact dermatitis. Note the hyperpigmentation affecting the perioral, periocular regions, in addition to the concave aspect of the pinna and the upper portion of the vertical ear canal.

Fig. 3.8 Allergic contact dermatitis following neomycin therapy. Erythematous, hyperplastic otitis externa. Note the lack of lesions on the concave aspect of the pinna, a pointer to this not being atopy, even though the changes in the external ear canal are indistinguishable on clinical grounds.

Autoimmune/immune mediated

> ### KEY POINT
>
> - Autoimmune and immune-mediated diseases rarely cause ear disease.

Where lesions include vesicles, bullae, ulcers, or erosions these diseases should be considered. Pemphigus foliaceus, pemphigus erythematosus, vasculitis, and systemic lupus erythematosus commonly affect the pinnae but very rarely cause otitis externa[1-4]. However, if vesicles, blisters, erosions, or ulcers are found on the concave aspect of the pinna and in the external ear canal (Figure 3.9), these diseases should be considered, particularly if bacteriology and cytology suggest minimal microbial involvement. Cytological examination of vesicular contents may reveal acanthocytes and neutrophils (see Figure 2.38), a combination suggestive of pemphigus foliaceus.

Ectoparasitic causes

- *Otodectes cynotis* is the most common ectoparasite involved in otitis externa.
- As few as three otodectic mites have been reported to cause otitis externa.
- Asymptomatic carriage of *O. cynotis* is common in the cat and may occur, though rarely, in the dog.
- *O. cynotis* may, very rarely, be zoonotic.
- Other ectoparasitic causes of otitis externa include *Demodex* spp., *Neotrombicula autumnalis* and other harvest mites, and ticks such as *Otobius megnini*.

Otodectes cynotis

O. cynotis (Figure 3.10) is a large (0.3–0.4 mm [0.01–0.02 in]) mite which lives predominantly in the external ear canal of dogs and cats, and perhaps occasionally on the adjacent skin of the head[1]. The mite does not burrow but lives on the skin surface where it feeds on tissue fluid and debris[2]. It has been suggested that otodectic mites can

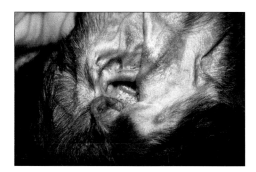

Fig. 3.9 Primary lesions of pemphigus foliaceus at the entrance to the external ear canal and on the concave aspect of the pinna. Cytological examination of samples taken from these lesions reveals neutrophils and 'rounded up' keratinocytes, called acanthocytes (see Fig. **2.38**).

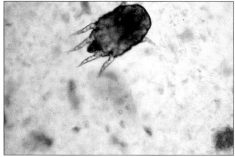

Fig. 3.10 Photomicrograph of an adult *Otodectes cynotis* mite.

survive within the household, off the host, for weeks if not months[3].

The physical presence of the mite induces a mechanical irritation which accounts for some of the pruritus experienced by infected animals. However, the saliva is both irritant and immunogenic and in the cat the mite stimulates an IgE-like antibody[2], suggesting that hypersensitivity contributes to the pruritus. The mite produces an antibody which cross-reacts with the house dust mite *Dermatophagoides farinae*[3] and may thus play a part in human atopy. Ear mite antigen may play a part in inducing aural haematoma in both the dog and cat and this might have an autoimmune aetiology[4,5].

Zoonotic lesions may occur on in-contact human members of the household[1]. Vesicles, wheals, erythematous papules, and excoriations on the arms and torso have been reported[6].

Lifecycle, transmission, and prevalence

Females lay eggs (Figure 3.11) and cement them to the epidermal surface. These hatch to yield six-legged larvae which undergo two moults through eight-legged protonymphs and deutonymphs. The emerging deutonymph is approached by, and attached to, an adult male mite (Figure 3.12) and, if it is female, copulation occurs. Although the life cycle of 3 weeks is confined to the host, it has been suggested that the mite can survive in the environment for long periods[3]. Nevertheless, contact with an infected host is still believed to be the main route of transmission[1].

The prevalence of *O. cynotis* in dogs' ears was assessed as 29.1% in one study of 700 ears, with a significant predisposition in dogs with pendulous and semierect pinnae as compared to erect pinnae[7]. This study also reported that there was a highly significant correlation between the presence of mites and otitis externa. In 114 (out of 700 ears) ears, mites were found in the absence of any indication of otitis externa, suggesting that in dogs, asymptomatic carriage is possible. Fewer cases were reported in the summer months. One study[8] suggested a seasonal incidence for the disease; however, a very large study[9] could find no evidence of a seasonal incidence. Note that many of these studies on the prevalence of *O. cynotis* were performed before the widespread use of topical and systemic ectoparasiticides.

Young dogs appear to be more commonly infected than older animals[9]. This probably reflects the fact that infected dogs are easily diagnosed, effectively treated, and not reinfected. The average number of mites per dog was only 5.6[9].

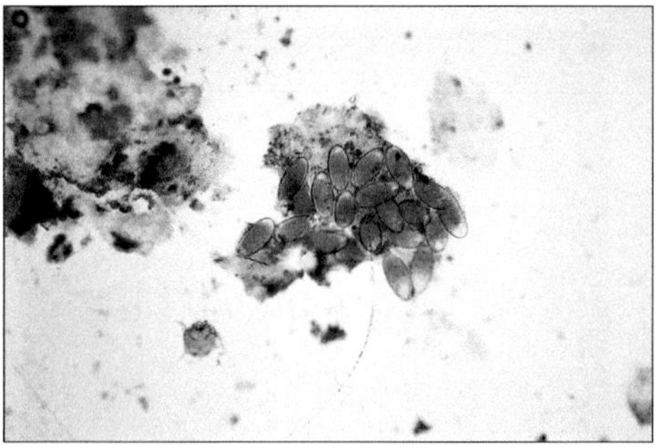

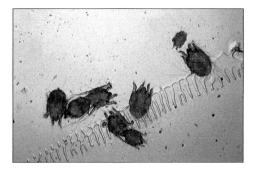

Fig. 3.11 Photomicrograph of *Otodectes* spp. ova collected in cerumen.

Fig. 3.12 Photomicrograph of two deutonymphs each attached to an adult otodectic mite.

Scott[8] suggested an age predilection in young cats. In cases of chronic infection there may be hyperplastic changes in the lining of the external ear canal and a predisposition to secondary infection.

Clinical features

O. cynotis is typically associated with a pruritic otitis externa[7,8]. However, Scott[8] considered that in the cat, three syndromes (otitis externa, ectopic infection, and asymptomatic carriage) might be associated with infection with the mite.

Very low numbers of mites, even as low as three[7], may be sufficient to induce clinical signs. This, together with the mite's ability to inhabit the entire external ear canal, can make definitive diagnosis difficult and might make a rule-out of otodectic acariasis, other than by trial therapy, problematic.

The classic feature of otitis externa due to ear mite infection is moderate to severe otic pruritus. In addition, the external ear canal becomes filled with a crumbly black/brown discharge (Figures 3.13–3.15). Most affected dogs exhibit chronic otic pruritus but Frost[7] reported four dogs out of 200 which had asymptomatic infection. Puppies are most likely to be infected from dams, but in adult dogs the cat is a common cause of contagion[1], particularly since the cat may well be asymptomatic[8,10].

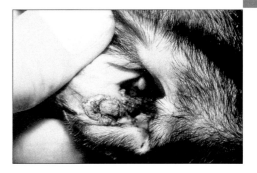

Fig. 3.13 Adult cat with *Otodectes cynotis* infestation. Note the typical dark brown colour and the dry nature of the cerumen. Note also the lack of self-trauma in this asymptomatic case.

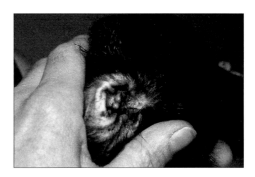

Fig. 3.14 Otodectic mange in a pup. Note the presence of the dryish cerumen and evidence of some self-trauma.

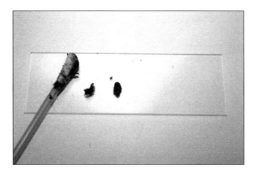

Fig. 3.15 Cerumen from an ear infested with *Otodectes cynotis*. Note the crumbly nature of the cerumen and the dark brown colour.

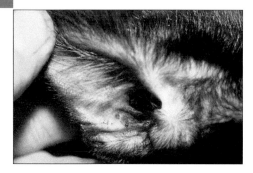

Fig. 3.16 Small area of crust and self-trauma in the entrance to the external ear canal of a cat with otodectic otitis.

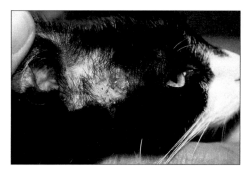

Fig. 3.17 Area of erythema and self-trauma associated with otodectic otitis on the lateral aspect of the head of a cat.

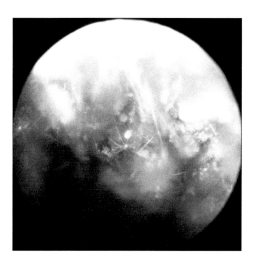

In cats the pruritus associated with infection may be associated with moderate to severe self-trauma to the head (Figures 3.16, 3.17).

In some cases, perhaps in cats more than in dogs, the mite causes clinical signs distant from the ear. Scott[8] considered that this might be a consequence of cats sleeping in a curled position so that the ear is apposed to the tail-base. Two syndromes may be associated with ectopic infection:
- Crusted papules, i.e. miliary dermatitis.
- Patchy alopecia.

Asymptomatic infection may be a feature of older cats where very high numbers of mites may be found with apparently no associated clinical signs[10]. The presence of asymptomatic carriage in dogs has not been considered a major problem in veterinary dermatological texts, but in light of the discussion above it should be borne in mind, particularly when treatment protocols are discussed.

Diagnosis

The mite is relatively large and may be easily seen in the external ear canal with the aid of an auroscope (Figure 3.18). Direct observation may not always result in a diagnosis:
- The degree of discharge may make direct observation difficult.
- There may be so few mites that direct observation is not possible.

In these situations, microscopic examination of discharge may be necessary. Gentle maceration of collected samples in mineral oil will aid diagnosis, and microscopic examination under low power should show evidence of infestation.

Fig. 3.18 Otoscopic view of ceruminous debris and otodectic mites in a feline external ear canal. The mites appear small in this unmagnified view.

Demodex canis, D. felis, and D. gatoi

Demodex canis has been reported as a rare cause of otitis externa in dogs. It may occur as part of a generalized condition, in isolation, or as a long-term complication of juvenile-onset generalized demodicosis which has apparently responded to treatment[11]. A history of demodicosis should alert the clinician to the possibility of otodemodicosis but cases arising *de novo* should not be discounted. Typically, otodemodicosis is associated with a ceruminous otitis externa (Figure 3.19).

In cats, demodicosis is more usually associated with erythema (Figure 3.20) and crusting on the pinnae and head, rather than otitis externa. However, *D. gatoi* may be associated with a ceruminous otitis externa in cats.

Diagnosis is based on recovery of demodecid mites (Figures 3.21–3.23) in skin scrapes and on cotton swabs from the external ear canal. Punch biopsy samples would also give appropriate material for a diagnosis.

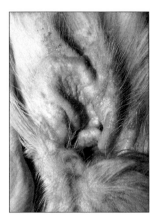
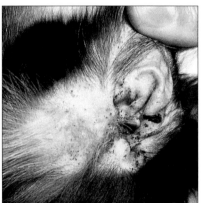

Fig. 3.19 Erythematous, ceruminous otitis externa in a Cavalier King Charles Spaniel with otodemodicosis.

Fig. 3.20 Feline demodicosis causing erythematous dermatitis adjacent to the entrance to the external ear canal.

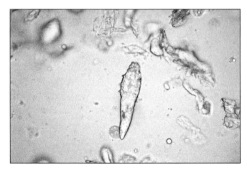
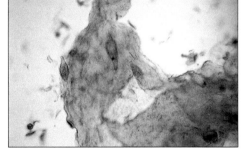

Figs. 3.21, 3.22 Photomicrographs of a juvenile demodectic mite (**3.21**) and an egg (**3.22**) in cerumen from the ear of a dog with otodemodectic mange.

Fig. 3.23 Photomicrograph of an adult *Demodex canis* mite in cerumen from the external ear canal of a dog with otodemodectic mange.

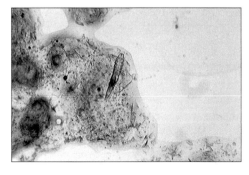

Harvest mites

Harvest mites, such as *Neotrombicula autumnalis* (Figure 3.24) and *Euotrombicula alfredugesi*, are occasional causes of otitis externa in both dogs and cats. The larvae are parasitic and require a mammalian host; they are not species specific. Larvae hatch in rapid succession and usually tens or hundreds are involved in the parasitic attack. Typically, they cause a pruritic crusting dermatitis on the ventrum and face and in the interdigital areas. Occasional animals exhibit larval clustering and crusting at the base of the pinnae[17] or within the confines of the proximal external ear canal. Close examination usually reveals tiny orange, or orange-red, clusters of larvae.

The parasite is a seasonal threat to the hunting or roaming dog and cat and it is more common on ground composed of well drained, chalky soil.

Ticks

The spinous ear tick, *Otobius megnini*, (Figure 3.25) is most frequently found in the southern and south-western regions of the USA. However, the increased mobility of owners and their pets means that the tick may be found in almost any region of the USA[13,14]. The larvae (six legs, yellow-pink colour) and adults (eight legs, blue-grey colour) are parasitic and infest the external ear canal of both dogs and cats to the extent that in some cases the external ear canal is entirely filled with the parasites. Acute otitis externa results. Ixodic, hard ticks such as *Demacentor* spp., and the rabbit 'stick tight flea' (*Spillopsyllus cuniculi*) are usually found on the pinnae and head, rather than within the external ear canal.

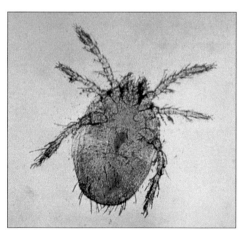

Fig. 3.24 Larva of *Neotrombicula autumnalis*. Note the red colour and six legs.

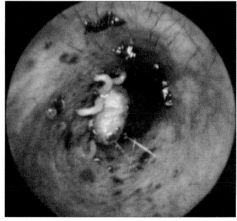

Fig. 3.25 *Otobius megnini* in the external ear canal of a dog. (Courtesy of Dr. Louis Gotthelf, DVM; Mongomery, AL, USA.)

Endocrinopathies

KEY POINT
■ Endocrine disease is an uncommon cause of otitis externa in the dog or cat.

Endocrinopathies are often cited as underlying causes of chronic ceruminous otitis externa. However, neither hypo-thyroidism nor hyperadrenocorticism are commonly associated with otitis externa[1–3]; allergy is a much more common cause. Hypothyroidism should be suspected as a cause in middle aged predisposed breeds (e.g. Labradors, Labrador Retrievers) when they present in middle age with no previous history of ear problems. Gonadal hormone changes (e.g. Sertoli cell tumours), in contrast, may have a profound effect on cutaneous glandular function and may therefore be associated with ceruminous otitis (Figure 3.26) in association with other signs[4].

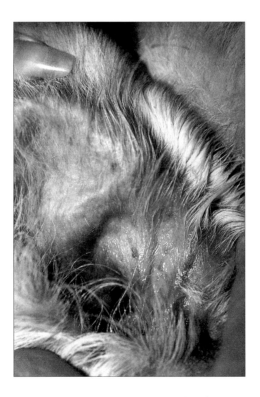

Fig. 3.26 Otitis externa associated with a Sertoli cell tumor. Note the ceruminous discharge adhering to the concave aspect of the pinna.

Epithelialization disorders

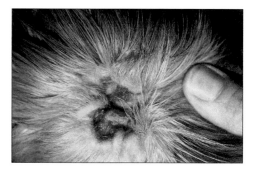

Fig. 3.27 Early changes associated with chronic otitis externa in a Cocker Spaniel. Ceruminous otitis with early hyperplasia.

Epithelialization disorders include seborrhoeic diseases which are caused by defects in keratinization, sebaceous adenitis, vitamin A responsive dermatosis, and zinc responsive dermatosis. Defects in keratinization may be primary or be secondary to another disease. By far the most common causes of scaling and crusting dermatoses are secondary causes such as ectoparasites, infectious agents, hypersensitivities, and endocrinopathies[2]. Otitis externa may be anticipated with these disorders only if the underlying disease is itself a cause of ear disease. Superficial pyoderma, dermatophytosis, or demodicosis are common causes of crust and scale on the trunk or limbs, but they rarely cause otitis externa. In contrast, the inflammation caused by atopy is generalized, as are the aberrations in cutaneous homeostasis which accompany an endocrinopathy. Thus, these diseases are often associated with otitis externa.

Similarly, some, but not all, of the primary defects in keratinization (idiopathic seborrhoea) may be associated with otitis externa. Examples include idiopathic seborrhoea in Cocker Spaniels[3] and epidermal dysplasia in West Highland White Terriers[4]. The relationship between epidermal dysplasia and the yeast *Malassezia pachydermatis* in West Highland White Terriers is complex and poorly understood[4,5]. Basset Hounds also suffer from a dermatosis which used to be classified as idiopathic seborrhoea. Many of these dogs suffer from *M. pachydermatis* dermatitis and they show a spectacular response to antimalassezial therapy[6]. Whatever the exact nature of these two disorders, or their relationship, they are both associated with severe otitis externa[4,6].

The otitis externa associated with primary seborrhoea in Cocker Spaniels is initially ceruminous (Figure 3.27), but epidermal hyperplasia (Figure 3.28) soon follows. The otic discharge is typically thick and oleaginous (Figure 3.29). Otoscopic examination of early cases reveals hyperplasia, a moister appearance than in an atopic ear canal (compare with Figures 3.1–3.3), and a tendency to bleed easily (Figure 3.30). Cytological examination from many cases will reveal plenty of cerumen and cellular debris but only a few inflammatory cells (Figure 3.31). Indeed, subsequent bacterial culture from

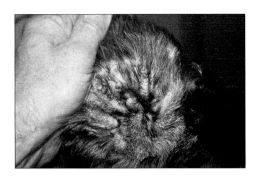

Fig. 3.28 Cocker Spaniel with an almost occluded external ear canal, a consequence of chronic otitis externa.

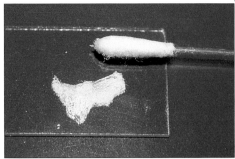

Fig. 3.29 Unstained cytology smear. Note the thick, oleaginous nature of the cerumen.

Fig. 3.30 Otoscopic picture of the external ear canal of a Cocker Spaniel with early changes associated with chronic otitis externa. There is erythema and the ear canal has a moister appearance than the atopic ear (compare with Figs. 3.1–3.3). Note that the ear canal has been plucked to facilitate cleaning.

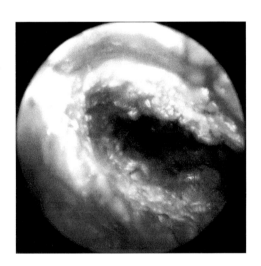

Fig. 3.31 Photomicrograph of a stained cytological smear from a Cocker Spaniel. Note the increased numbers of squames, the amount of cerumen, the lack of micro-organisms, and the absence of inflammatory cells.

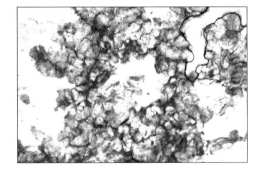

these ears may fail to record any significant bacterial growth at all, illustrating the value of otic cytology. However, in contrast to the otitis associated with atopy, the disease in Cocker Spaniels is often complicated by gram-negative infection (Figure 3.32), perhaps a reflection of differences in glandular secretion.

Hereditary defects in keratinization have been reported in cats[1]. Persian cats are most commonly affected (Figure 3.33), although the condition may occur in other breeds. Affected animals show signs from a very early age and either sex may be affected. The ears develop a ceruminous otitis externa and greasy scale may accumulate on the pinnae. The entire trunk is also affected with scale, grease, and malodour. Because of the severity of the disease, many cases are euthanazed at an early age as there is no effective treatment.

Foreign bodies

KEY POINTS

- Younger dogs from hunting and working breeds are predisposed.
- Otic foreign bodies usually, but not always, cause acute clinical signs of otitis.
- Always examine both ears as foreign bodies may be bilateral.
- Grass awns are the most common foreign body entering the external ear canal.
- Rupture of the tympanum is a common complication of otic foreign body penetration.
- Otic foreign bodies are most commonly seen in the summer, reflecting the importance of grass awns in the aetiology.

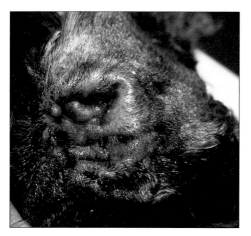

Fig. 3.32 Ulcerated external ear canal due to gram-negative bacterial infection in a Cocker Spaniel.

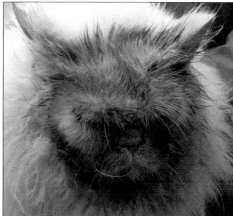

Fig. 3.33 Persian cat with an hereditary defect in keratinization. There is a greasy otitis externa.

There is no sex predisposition to otic foreign body penetration but young dogs are predisposed to grass awn penetration[1,2]. In general, all breeds of Spaniels and Golden Retrievers are most commonly affected, while German Shepherd Dogs, Miniature Poodles, and Dachshunds are under-represented[2].

The most common foreign body found in the external ear canal of dogs and cats is the grass awn[1]. In the USA the most common species of plant awn is *Hordeum jubatum*, although other members of the genus, such as *H. murinum*, *H. silvestre*, and genera such as *Stipa*, *Setaria*, *Bromus*, and *Avena*, may be involved in other areas of the world[2]. All have a similar shape (Figure 3.34) with wiry barbs which prevent retrograde movement; once in the ear canal they can only move forward (Figure 3.35).

Hair shafts, particularly if they contact the tympanum, may also act as foreign bodies (Figure 3.36). In one series of 120 cases of otitis externa, 12.6% of the cases were considered to result from matted hair and cerumen in the external ear canal[3]. Other foreign bodies that may enter, or be put into, the external ear canal include other

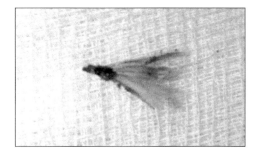

Fig. 3.34 Typical shape of a grass awn; this was removed from the external ear canal of a dog.

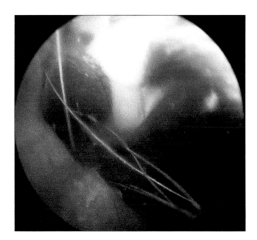

Fig. 3.35 Otoscopic picture of a grass awn lying adjacent to the tympanic membrane. In this case the grass awn had not punctured the tympanum; however, note the area of erythema and erosion on the tympanic membrane.

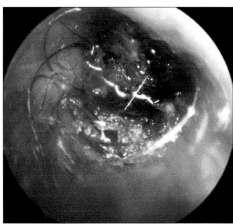

Fig. 3.36 Accumulation of hair and cerumen obstructing the horizontal ear canal at the level of the tympanum.

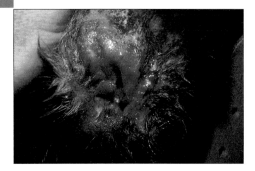

Fig. 3.37 Acute, erythematous, ulcerated otitis externa associated with the penetration of a grass awn into the external ear canal.

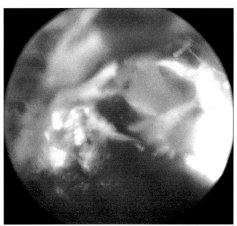

Fig. 3.38 Grass awn penetration of the tympanum. Note the small piece of vegetation still visible on the left, adjacent to the area of haemorrhage.

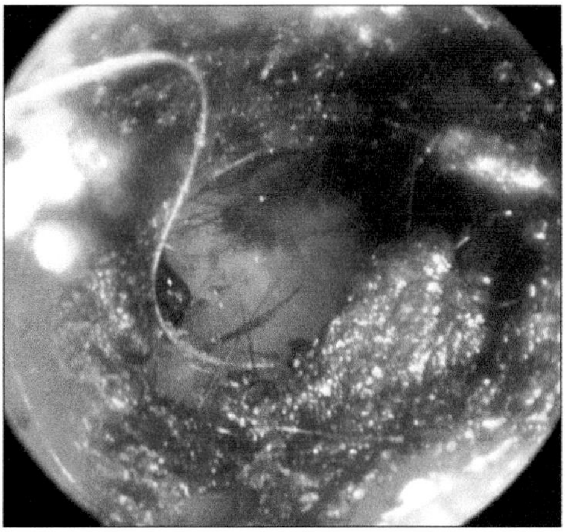

Fig. 3.39 Grass awn penetration, picture taken with video-otoscope, note the increase in clarity and depth of field.

pieces of vegetation and children's toys. Aggregations of otic, usually proprietary, nonveterinary powders and ointments with cerumen may also induce foreign body reactions. Occasionally a clinician is presented with a young dog exhibiting acute otic discomfort. Examination reveals no evidence of ear disease and no foreign bodies are found. It may be that the dog's violent shaking has dislodged the accumulation of cerumen that was the cause of the irritation.

Foreign body penetration into the ear canal is usually accompanied by acute pain. The dog or cat shakes its head and may attempt to remove the object with a foot. As the object moves down it may induce hyperaemia and ulceration followed by the generation of an otic discharge and secondary bacterial proliferation (Figure 3.37). If the foreign body penetrates the epithelial lining of the external ear canal, it may become embedded in a pyogranuloma[4]. In one study[2] nearly 20% of cases of otic grass awn penetration were associated with rupture of the tympanum (Figures 3.38, 3.39), suggesting that otitis media should be considered in long-standing cases, even where the tympanum is intact.

The most common bacteria associated with grass awns are streptococci, although *Staphylococcus* spp, *Pasteurella* spp., and *Actinomycetes* spp. may also be cultured[2].

SECONDARY CAUSES OF OTITIS EXTERNA

KEY POINTS

- The bacterial flora of the canine external ear canal is principally a gram-positive flora, similar to that of the interfollicular epidermis.
- The vertical portion of the external ear canal contains more bacteria than the horizontal portion.
- Not all external ear canals contain significant numbers of bacteria or yeast.
- Otic inflammation is accompanied initially by an increase in the number of bacteria and a shift towards coagulase-positive staphylococci.
- Chronic inflammation in dogs is accompanied by increased numbers of gram-negative bacteria.
- *Malassezia pachydermatis* is regarded as an opportunistic pathogen.
- Otitis media may be present in over 80% of cases of otitis externa.
- The bacterial flora in the inner ear may be different from that of the external ear.

Microbiological changes associated with otitis externa

The overall changes in bacterial flora associated with otitis externa are qualitative and quantitative (*Table 3.2*); the number of bacteria increases and the proportion of various species changes (compare *Tables 3.1* and *3.2*). The incidence of recovery of staphylococci in general, and of coagulase-positive staphylococci in particular, increases[1-3]. More particularly, the incidence of recovery of *Pseudomonas* spp. and *Proteus* spp. increases[4-18].

Early studies[1] reported that *Proteus* spp. and *Pseudomonas* spp. were commonly isolated from certain breeds of dog, particularly the Cocker Spaniel, but not

recovered from others, such as the Miniature Poodle. The authors postulated that Miniature Poodles presented with acute, painful ear disease with a short time course, whereas Cocker Spaniels were notorious for exhibiting chronic otitis externa, permitting contamination with gram-negative organisms.

A more rational explanation is that Cocker Spaniels are anatomically prone to narrow, hirsute ear canals and to defects in keratinization. Both of these factors are likely to predispose to chronic otitis externa and gram-negative bacterial infection, particularly if the humidity within the external ear canal is elevated because of a pendulous pinna.

Miniature Poodles, on the other hand, might well have hirsute canals but they are often affected by atopy. Atopy is associated with an inflamed, erythematous otitis, at least at first, which is not exudative. Such changes mimic those on the skin and might be sufficiently aberrant to favour colonization by *Staphylococcus pseudintermedius* and *M. pachydermatis*, but not *P. aeruginosa*. Support for this contention comes from a Brazilian study in which the microbial flora of dogs with only bilateral otitis externa was studied[19]. The most frequent organisms isolated were *Staphylococcus intermedius* and *M. pachydermatis* – exactly what would be expected if the population contained a large number of allergic dogs, who typically manifest bilateral otitis externa.

The most common bacteria recovered from otitis externa in cats' ears were coagulase-positive staphylococci (54.8%). Gram-negative bacteria, such as *Pseudomonas* spp. and *Proteus* spp., were only rarely recovered from feline otitis externa[8].

M. pachydermatis is a yeast-like fungus commonly isolated from both normal and diseased external ear canals of dogs and cats. The number of organisms recovered varies, as does the rate of recovery of the yeast from ear canals. Thus recovery rates of between 14.3% and 37% have been reported for healthy dogs[3–8,20]. There appears to be the same environmental effect on the carriage of *M. pachydermatis* in normal ears as there is on gram-negative bacteria, with a higher rate of recovery in tropical and subtropical regions compared to temperate areas. Currently, the organism is regarded as an opportunist pathogen, capable of causing inflammatory changes in the ear canal, at least in the presence of moisture[21]. This is not to minimize its importance as a potentiator of chronic, or acute, otic inflammation, but it serves to suggest to the clinician that a search for underlying causes of the inflammation should be made. *M. pachydermatis* is a common cause of otitis externa in West Highland White Terriers and Basset Hounds. In these animals the ears are erythematous, malodorous, and hyperplastic (Figures 3.40, 3.41). Cerumen may be thick and oleaginous and vast numbers of yeast may be detected when smears are stained and examined microscopically (Figure 3.42).

The fungal flora of the ear canal also changes in otitis externa (*Tables 3.1* and *3.2*) and almost all of the increase results from an increased incidence of *M. pachydermatis*. Thus, Fraser[10] recovered *M. pachydermatis* from 36% of normal ear canals and from 44% of cases of otitis externa. However, the incidence of fungi was unchanged; indeed the number of isolations of *Aspergillus* spp., *Penicillium* spp., and *Rhizopus* spp. was reduced in otitic ear canals.

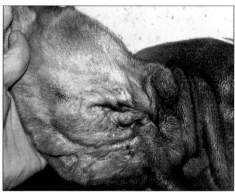

Fig. 3.41 Greasy, erythematous, malodorous, hyperplastic otitis externa in a Bassett Hound. Note the extension of the lesions on the pinna.

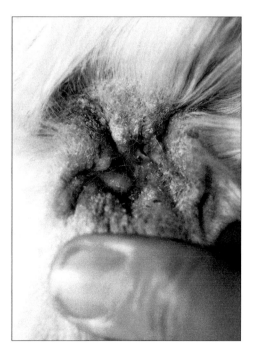

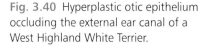

Fig. 3.40 Hyperplastic otic epithelium occluding the external ear canal of a West Highland White Terrier.

PERPETUATING FACTORS

KEY POINTS

- Pathological changes within the external ear canal are progressive.
- Changes in structure engender changes in the local microenvironment.
- Surgery is the inevitable consequence of chronic otitis externa.

Response to insult and injury
Reactions to inflammation within the external ear canal

The epidermis of the external ear canal reacts to inflammation by increasing its rate of turnover and increasing in thickness, i.e. it becomes hyperplastic[1,2]. There may be surface erosions and ulceration, particularly with gram-negative infections. The dermis becomes infiltrated with inflammatory cells and fibrosis will follow. In the early stages of otitis externa there is hyperplasia of the sebaceous glands, and their ducts may become dilated[3,4]. If chronic otitis persists, the apocrine glands become hyperplastic with cystic dilatation of the glands and ducts. Although this may be of such magnitude that the sebaceous glands appear displaced, with very little secretory potential[1,2], morphometric analysis reveals no significant changes in sebaceous gland size or activity[4]. Papillary proliferation of ceruminous glands and ducts may obliterate the lumen of the external ear canal in some cases[2]. In very chronic cases, ossification of the tissues may take place.

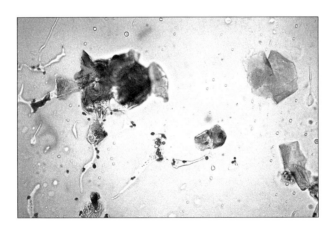

Fig. 3.42 Cytological smear demonstrating cerumen, squames, and many yeast.

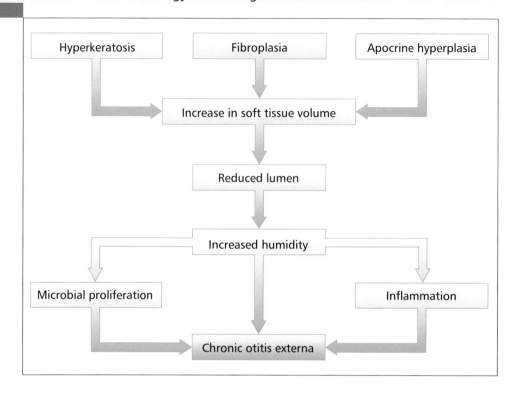

Fig. 3.43 Flow chart summarizing the progression of otitis externa.

Similar changes take place in the feline ear canal, although the papillary changes in the ceruminous glands may be sufficiently florid that discrete polyps occur[2].

The consequence of these changes is a reduction in luminal cross-section, a result of increasing soft tissue within the bounds of the containing cartilage[5]. The change in nature of the cerumen, the reduction in luminal diameter, and the moisture and warmth which accompany active inflammation contribute to an increase in local humidity[5]. These changes in the otic environment result in surface maceration and the creation of a milieu favourable to microbial multiplication, itself a potent inducer of inflammation (Figure 3.43).

It is not clear at which stage these changes become irreversible. Certainly, aggressive medical therapy, initially with antimicrobial agents and then with topical glucocorticoids, can result in significant reduction in soft tissue occlusion of the lumen. However, the structural changes in apocrine ducts and glands are probably irreversible; certainly the progressive changes in glandular architecture correlate with the progression of the otitis externa[4].

Even very early changes in the luminal epithelia have the potential to become permanent and, once these permanent changes occur, simple Zepp resection of the lateral wall of the vertical canal is unlikely to be successful[6-8]. Ablation of the canal is indicated.

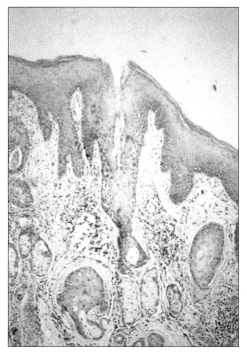

Fig. 3.44 Photomicrograph of a section of canine external ear canal demonstrating epidermal hyperplasia.

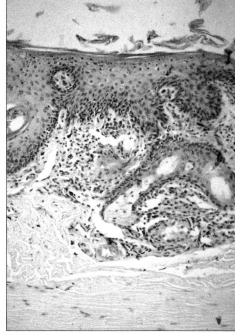

Fig. 3.45 Photomicrograph of a section of canine external ear canal demonstrating epidermal hyperplasia, an inflammatory infiltrate, and dermal oedema.

Influence of progressive pathology

The soft tissues surrounding the lumen of the external ear canal react in a predictable sequence to the inflammation associated with chronic otitis externa[1-4]:

- Epidermal hyperplasia (acanthosis and hyperkeratinization) is an early consequence of otic irritation (Figure 3.44). The basal cells of the epidermis respond to inflammation by increasing their rate of division and increasing the transit time of cells moving through the epidermis. In addition, keratinization is affected and a thickened stratum corneum is apparent. This reaction is reversible, provided the initiating cause is alleviated.

- Subepithelial infiltration with inflammatory cells, such as lymphocytes, neutrophils, macrophages, and plasma cells, occurs in response to inflammation. Chronic cellular infiltration results in local release of inflammatory mediators, cutaneous erythema, and oedema (Figure 3.45). Early cellular infiltration is reversible but the effects of chronic mediator release may engender permanent changes.

- Fibroplasia of the underlying dermis follows chronic inflammatory challenge within the lumen and the epithelium. In long-standing cases the fibrosis may be extensive (Figure 3.46), and this contributes considerably to the loss of luminal cross-section.
- Early sebaceous gland hyperplasia is followed by massive ceruminous gland hyperplasia, both of the duct and the glandular portion (Figure 3.47). The changes in the ceruminous glands result in gross thickening of the epidermis, particularly in cats.
- Papillary proliferation of the epithelial lining occurs to such an extent that the lumen becomes occluded (Figures 3.48, 3.49). In the external ear canals of cats this papillary proliferation may result in polyp formation, with trapping of exudate between the polyp and the tympanum.
- Ossification of the dermis, sometimes extending to the auricular cartilage, occurs as a final stage.

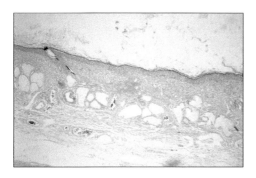

Fig. 3.46 Photomicrograph of a section of canine external ear canal stained to demonstrate dermal fibrosis, which in this case is extensive.

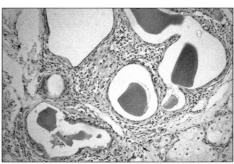

Fig. 3.47 Photomicrograph of a section of canine external ear canal demonstrating massive apocrine gland hyperplasia.

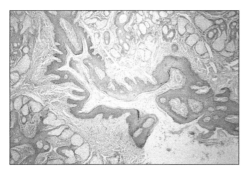

Fig. 3.48 Photomicrograph of a section of hyperplastic external ear canal with papillary fronds almost occluding the lumen.

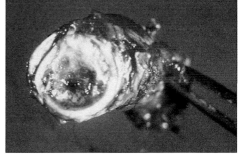

Fig. 3.49 Photograph of a section of a chronically hyperplastic external ear canal with almost no lumen.

Influence of breed

KEY POINTS

- Breeds of dog predisposed to otitis externa, such as Cocker Spaniels, have increased amounts of glandular tissue compared to normal dogs.
- Otitis externa results in increased production of cerumen with a lower lipid content than normal, associated with increased ceruminous gland activity.
- Conformational factors that may predispose to the development of otitis externa include dogs with stenotic ear canals, pendulous pinnae, hirsute pinnae, and hairy canals.

Fernando[1] observed that the external ear canals of longhaired breeds of dogs and those with fine hair contained more sebaceous and apocrine glandular tissue, which was also better developed, than dogs with short hair. Breeds predisposed to otitis externa also have abnormal morphometric ratios compared to normal dogs[2]. Specifically, they exhibit an increase in the overall amount of soft tissue within the confines of the auricular cartilage, an increase in the area occupied by the apocrine glands, and an increase in the apocrine gland area compared to that of the sebaceous glands.

Overall, the breeds of dog predisposed to otitis externa have increased apocrine tissue[2]. If this increased volume of apocrine tissue is actively secreting, the concentration of lipid within the cerumen will fall[3], humidity within the ear canal will rise, and maceration, followed by infection and otitis externa, will result. Increased moisture and surface maceration creates an environment particularly favourable to gram-negative bacteria. Theoretically, the increased apocrine secretions in the ear canals of these dogs should result in cerumen with a lower pH than normal and an environment not conducive to gram-negative colonization. It may be that the acidifying effect of increased ceruminous gland secretion is not sufficient to overcome the effects of humidity, inflammation, and surface maceration.

Dogs with pendulous ears are predisposed to otitis externa[1,3,4] but the low incidence in some breeds with pendulous ears, such as Beagles and Irish Setters, in most studies[1,2] suggests factors other than conformation at work. The presence of hair, *per se*, within the ear canal does not correlate with otitis externa[4]. However, Cocker Spaniels have many compound hair follicles throughout the length of the external ear canal whereas nonpredisposed breeds typically have fewer, predominantly simple follicles in their ear canals[5]. Certain breeds, such as Cocker Spaniels and Miniature Poodles, appear on every list of affected breeds[1,3, 5–8]. However, it is now recognized that one of the principal causes of otitis externa is the presence of hypersensitivities, such as atopy, and generalized skin disease, such as defects in keratinization, which predispose to otitis externa. It is the predisposition to these diseases which accounts for the increased relative risk of ear disease rather than the anatomy *per se*.

Only one study has recorded the incidence of otitis externa in cats. In this series of 36 cats, Himalayans and Persian breeds were most commonly affected[9].

Excessive moisture

> ### KEY POINTS
>
> - Increases in environmental temperature and humidity are reflected in the external ear canal.
> - The incidence of otitis externa peaks in late summer and early autumn.
> - Gram-negative infections of the external ear canal are more common in humid and warm environments.
> - Dogs that swim are also predisposed to developing signs of otitis externa.

The three main components of weather which impact on external ear disease are temperature, humidity, and rainfall. All three factors interact with each other and affect the internal environment of the external ear canal[1,2]. Thus, increasing environmental temperature or relative humidity is reflected in a small but measurable increase in temperature or relative humidity within the external ear canal[1]. The incidence of otitis externa increases as environmental temperature, relative humidity, and rainfall increases, although there is a lag effect of 1–2 months[3]. This results in a peak incidence of otitis externa, in dogs in late summer and early autumn[3].

Variations in climate, commensurate upon geographic location, affect both the incidence and type of otitis externa. Thus, although temperature, relative humidity, and rainfall all affect the incidence of otitis externa, the local climate also exerts an effect[3].

The local climate will also affect the microbial flora of the external ear canal. In hot and humid environments there are fewer ear canals from which no bacterial growth can be cultured[4]. In man the incidence of gram-negative bacterial complication of otitis externa increases in hot humid environments[5] and there is evidence that this is also the case in dogs[4].

Finally, in man it has been demonstrated that the incidence of asthma increases after thunderstorms[6]. Thunderstorms are associated with a decrease in temperature and an increase in humidity and rainfall and, more significantly, a significant rise in the concentration of pollen allergen in the air, secondary to osmotic rupture of pollen grains[7]. Given that a high proportion of cases of otitis externa are a consequence of atopy, it may be that some cases of acute otitis externa may also be related to thunderstorms.

Obstructive disease
Conchal neoplasia

> ### KEY POINTS
>
> - Neoplasia of the canine and feline external ear canal is rare.
> - Canine tumours are more likely to be benign, feline tumours are more likely to be malignant.
> - The most common benign tumours in the dog are papillomas, basal cell carcinomas, and ceruminous gland adenomas; in the cat ceruminous gland adenomas are the most common.
> - The most common malignant tumours in the dog and cat are carcinomas, adenocarcinomas, and squamous cell carcinomas.

Neoplasia of the external ear canal is rare[1]. In general, otic neoplasia in cats tends to be malignant[1,2] and is likely to be found in either the vertical or the horizontal canal with equal frequency[1]. Otic discharge, pruritus, and pain are common, whereas neurological signs are rare[1]. Canine conchal neoplasia is more likely to be benign than feline conchal neoplasia, but distribution and clinical signs are similar[1,2]. Most benign tumours do not affect the bullae[1]. Although the malignant tumours, particularly in the cat, tend to invade locally, it appears that distant metastasis is the exception rather than the rule[1]. When nervous signs accompany otic neoplasia, a generally poor prognosis is necessary since this usually indicates middle ear involvement and squamous cell carcinoma; altogether a more malignant tumour than ceruminous gland adenocarcinoma of the external ear canal[1]. Indeed, when squamous cell carcinoma is found in the external ear canal it usually has its origins in the middle ear.

Papillomas, basal cell tumours, and ceruminous gland adenomas are the most commonly found benign tumours in dogs, while in cats ceruminous gland adenomas are most common[1]. Carcinomas, adenocarcinomas, and squamous cell carcinomas are the most common malignant tumours in both dogs and cats. The clinical appearance of these neoplasms is usually that of a raised, frequently ulcerated mass which may occlude the lumen[3].

Ceruminous gland adenoma

Benign ceruminous gland neoplasia tends to present with signs of obstructive otitis externa (Figure 3.50): pruritus, head shaking, malodour, otorrhoea, and occasional haemorrhage[3,4]. Ceruminous gland adenomas are most commonly seen in middle-aged to elderly animals[4,5]. These benign tumours tend to be raised and occasionally pedunculated (Figure 3.51) and they may occlude the external ear canal[6]. They may have a melanotic appearance (Figure 3.52) and may be multiple[5]. Aggressive surgical management is usually curative and lateral wall resection, vertical wall ablation, or total ablation of the external ear canal is indicated, as dictated by the extent of the tumour.

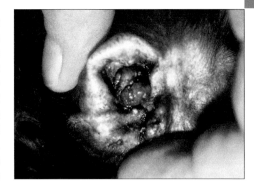

Fig. 3.50 Obstructive otitis secondary to ceruminous gland neoplasia in a cat.

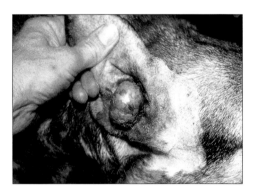

Fig. 3.51 Large, pedunculated ceruminous gland adenoma protruding from the external ear canal of a dog.

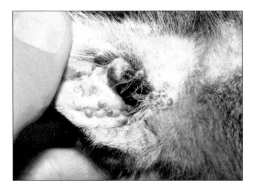

Fig. 3.52 Multiple, melanotic ceruminous gland adenomas in the external ear canal of a cat.

Ceruminous gland adenocarcinoma

Malignant ceruminous gland tumours tend to be ulcerative and infiltrating rather than occlusive[4,5]. Most cases tend to occur in old animals – cats: mean age 12 years; dogs: mean age 9 years[7,8]. Otoscopically they are pinkish in colour (Figure 3.53), ulcerated, and friable in nature[7,8]. Most dogs and cats exhibit an otic discharge which is commonly malodorous, purulent (Figure 3.54), and blood stained[7,8]. Otic pruritus and ipsilateral mandibular lymphadenopathy is also commonly noted[7,8]. Bulla involvement was demonstrated in nearly half the cats and dogs in recent studies[7,8]. This tendency to involve the bulla (Figures 3.55, 3.56) is reflected in the response to surgery: radical, total ear canal ablation and bulla osteotomy results in a longer disease-free interval, a lower recurrence rate, and longer postoperative survival time than simple lateral wall resection[7,8]. If the tumour has extended through the external ear canal into surrounding soft tissue, adjunctive radiotherapy is indicated[7,9].

Squamous cell carcinoma

In cats, squamous cell carcinoma appears to be as common as ceruminous gland adenocarcinoma[1]. The tumours are proliferative and ulcerated (Figure 3.57) and they have a tendency to grow rapidly[5]. Most conchal tumours with otoscopically visible evidence of extensive spread and histopathological evidence of local infiltration are squamous cell carcinomas[1]. Radical resection is necessary and presurgical biopsy may be advantageous.

Non neoplastic growths

Pyogenic granulomas

These have been reported to occur within the external ear canal of cats[10]. Clinically the granulomas appear as fleshy masses that may be covered in epithelium. However, the epithelial surface is usually ulcerated[10]. The prognosis for pyogenic granuloma is much better than for overt neoplasia. However, histopathological examination of biopsy samples is essential to distinguish the two.

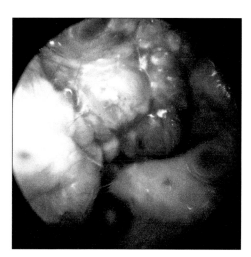

Fig. 3.53 Pinkish, nodular appearance of a ceruminous gland adenocarcinoma in the external ear canal of a cat.

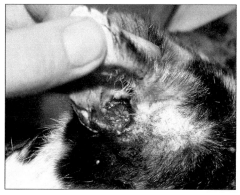

Fig. 3.54 Malodorous, haemorrhagic obstructive otitis secondary to ceruminous gland adenocarcinoma in a cat. The ulcerated mass of tumour may be seen protruding into the lumen at the entrance to the external ear canal.

Eosinophilic granulomas

Eosinophilic granuloma of the external ear canal has been reported in four dogs[11]. These dogs presented with chronic otitis externa. Otoscopic examination revealed a solitary, friable mass occluding the vertical canal. Surgical excision was curative.

Cryptococcosis

Cryptococcosis and other fungal disease may occasionally cause granulomatous lesions near the external ear canal (Figure 3.58). Histopathological examination of biopsy samples will identify these lesions. Cryptococcosis has a better prognosis than squamous cell carcinoma, thereby justifying biopsy.

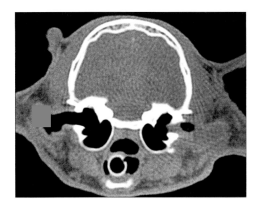

Fig. 3.55 CT scan of a 13-year-old cat. There is increased soft tissue opacity in the right external ear canal extending up to, and perhaps across, the tympanic membrane. This is a ceruminous gland adenocarcinoma. Note that the right bulla appears as normal as the left. The bony septum dividing the feline bulla into lateral and medial compartments is clearly visible with this imaging modality.

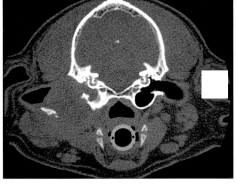

Fig. 3.56 CT scan of a 10-year-old Cocker Spaniel. The left-hand side exhibits an irregular, imprecise outline to the bulla, increased density within the bulla, loss of air within the external ear canal, mineralization of soft tissue in the external ear canal, and a homogenous soft tissue mass on the ventral aspect of the skull. This is a ceruminous gland adenocarcinoma.

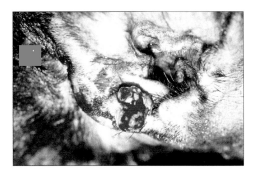

Fig. 3.57 Ulcerated, poorly-defined squamous cell carcinoma at the entrance to the external ear canal of a dog.

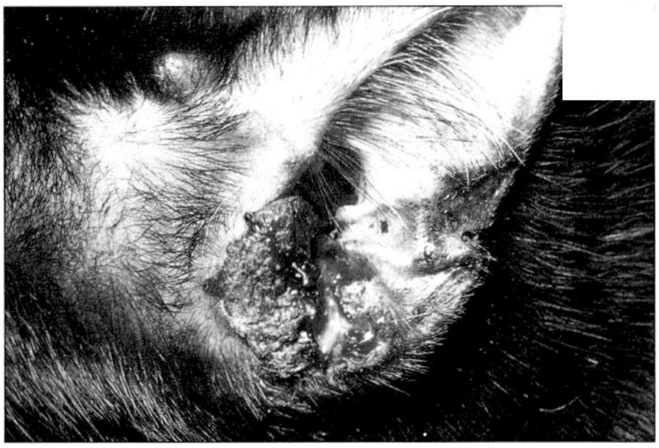

Fig. 3.58 Ulcerated granulomatous lesions due to cryptococcosis should be considered in the differential diagnosis of conchal neoplasia.

INTRODUCTION

KEY POINTS

- The integrity of the tympanum must be established before anything other than water or saline is put into the external ear canal.
- Many of the commonly used ceruminolytics exhibit ototoxic effects in the middle ear.
- Aural lavage and subsequent drying are the key steps in cleaning the external ear canal.
- Chemical depilation and ceruminolytics/ceruminosolvents may be an aid to cleaning the ear canal.

Inflamed ear canals contain increased amounts of moisture, aberrant cerumen, mucous, increased numbers of micro-organisms, and increased concentrations of microbial toxins. Foreign bodies, neo-plasms, or ectoparasites may be present. There may be inflammatory cells in the lumen, an inflammatory reaction within the epithelium, and erosions, or even ulceration, of the epithelium. The animal may well be showing signs of pain. The tympanum may be ruptured.

Aural lavage is beneficial for several reasons (after Little[1] and McKeever[2]):

- It removes exudate, debris, macerated epithelial components, micro-organisms, toxins, and some foreign bodies.
- It improves visualization of the proximal external ear canal and allows otoscopic examination of the deeper regions.
- It may permit visualization of the tympanum.
- It facilitates subsequent therapy.
- It may provide relief from pain.

The procedure for cleaning the external ear is straightforward and involves a number of distinct steps:

- Establish the integrity of the tympanum. If this cannot be assessed, use cleaning agents with a high degree of middle ear safety.
- Assess the discharge both visually and cytologically to decide if a flush or ceruminolytic/ceruminosolvent is most appropriate.
- Assess the canal to decide if a neutral/alkaline or acid cleaner is appropriate and whether a cleaner with antibacterial or antiyeast activity may be beneficial.
- Remove as much free fluid and discharge as possible with suction or very gentle swabbing.
- Apply a drying agent if possible to ensure complete removal of moisture.

ASSESSING THE INTEGRITY OF THE TYMPANUM

This step is critical since many cleaning techniques advocate chemicals and some degree of water pressure to flush the external ear canal. Any damage to the tympanum puts the middle and inner ear at risk[3].

Visual assessment of the tympanum is difficult in normal circumstances and often impossible when otitis externa is present. A variety of different techniques have been described to assess the tympanum. One includes filling the canal with warm water and watching to see if bubbles rise, another suggests the instillation of warm dilute povidone–iodine or dilute fluorescein into the canal and looking to see if fluid appears at the back of the throat or down the nose.

Auditory tympanometry, computed tomography or magnetic resonance imaging are advanced diagnostic techniques that may also be useful but are only really available in referral institutions. However Griffin[4] described a simple technique which allows indirect assessment of the tympanum. An otoscope is used to visualize the distal horizontal canal. A small, soft rubber feeding tube is passed through the otoscope toward the tympanum. If it continues to pass unhindered, the tympanum is ruptured or there is false middle ear syndrome. If its progress is blocked and the tip remains in view, the tympanum is intact. Assessing the tympanum with a Spreull needle is not advised since such a needle has the potential to rupture the tympanum.

ASSESSING THE DISCHARGE

Although there are of course exceptions to the rule, different disease processes tend to produce consistent changes in the appearance of the external ear canal and in the type of discharge. Assessment of the discharge allows selection of the most appropriate type of ear cleaner (Figure 4.1). Where the discharge is thick and waxy, as is often the case in keratinization disorders, endocrine disease,

Type of discharge	Dark brown	Pale brown	Yellow	Green
	Thick waxy	Moderate waxy purulent	Mild waxy purulent	Purulent haemorrhagic mucoid
Typical findings	Ceruminous otitis	Malassezial otitis	Staphylococcal otitis	Pseudomonal otitis
The waxier the discharge the more important the ceruminolytic property of the cleaner				
Ceruminolytic activity				
The more purulent and mucoid the discharge the higher the water content of the cleaner should be to flush the ear				
Flushing activity				

Fig. 4.1 Chart for the assessment of discharge.

and in allergy in such breeds as the Cocker Spaniel, then the cleaner needs to have the ability to break up the wax. Such cleaners need potent ceruminolytic or ceruminosolvent (oil-based lubricant) activity. Where the discharge is more purulent or mucopurulent in bacterial infection, especially where there is gram-negative infection and/or concurrent otitis media, then an aqueous-based flush is most appropriate.

Ceruminolytics and ceruminosolvents

Clinicians should be aware of the difference between a true ceruminolytic and a lubricant or ceruminosolvent:

- A ceruminolytic disrupts the integrity of cerumen by inducing lysis of the squames[5].
- A ceruminosolvent merely softens and loosens the cerumen.

Many authors[2,4,6–8] advocate an initial application of ceruminolytic agents prior to lavage in cases of otitis externa. The justification for this is that the action of the ceruminolytic, and some of the additives which may potentiate their effect, softens the ceruminous debris and cerumenocellular aggregates, permitting easy removal with subsequent aural lavage.

Ceruminolysis is optimal in hypo-osmolar, alkaline solutions[5]. Proteins on the surface of squames dissolve into this alkaline solution, binding with free hydroxyl ions. Loss of surface proteins reduces the integrity of the cell membrane and water enters the cell, resulting in swelling and fragmentation[5]. Disruption of the squames results in disintegration of the cerumen, allowing it to be flushed from the external ear canal.

A study on commercially available ceruminolytics[3] demonstrated that glycerine-based ceruminolytics, including carbamide peroxide/dioctyl sulfosuccinate and triethanolamine polypeptide oleate-condensate preparations, were ototoxic

(vestibular effects) and caused inflammatory changes within the middle ear. It was not clear which component(s) of the various products was/were responsible for the changes. In the same study the ceruminosolvent squalene was shown not to have any ototoxic effects.

No *in vivo* or *in vitro* studies have been performed on canine or feline cerumen. However, studies on human cerumen demonstrated that aqueous alkaline solutions of sodium hydroxide (0.1 molar), sodium bicarbonate (0.5% and 1.25%), and sodium dodecyl sulphate (0.05% and 0.1%) were superior to organic agents such as glycerine, triethanolamine polypeptide oleate-condensate, and olive oil[5]. Proprietary oil-based ceruminolytics were found to be no better than glycerine or olive oil.

None of the oil-based products had any true ceruminolytic effect; all merely lubricated and softened the bolus of cerumen[5,9]. However, softening and lubricating may be just as useful as true ceruminolysis since a blind, controlled study[10] failed to show significant differences between sterile water, sodium bicarbonate solution, and a lipid-based proprietary 'ceruminolytic'.

Water-based proprietary ceruminolytic preparations usually possess surfactant and emulsifying properties which allow aqueous substances to penetrate and under-run oily masses. These are preferred to oil-based products for two reasons:

- Firstly, they are less messy[7] and are more easily removed from the ear canal, permitting quicker cleaning and drying.
- Secondly, oil-based preparations are occlusive and may, if not thoroughly removed, potentiate bacterial infections[8].

Dioctyl sodium sulfosuccinate and calcium sulfosuccinate are effective emulsifiers[11] but they must not be used in dogs or cats if there is a ruptured tympanum[3,4]. Carbamate peroxide is a less potent agent than the sulfosuccinates[4] but is still capable of damaging the middle ear[3]. The foaming effect of released urea and oxygen may help to loosen adhered debris. This product is probably most useful in cases of purulent otitis externa[4].

Oil-based proprietary ceruminosolvents have a lubricant, diluting effect, permitting subsequent flushing out. Squalene, tri-ethanolamine polypeptide oleate-condensate, and hexamethyltetracosane are more potent than propylene glycol and mineral oil, but are not as powerful as the aqueous products detailed above which have a powerful surfactant activity[4]. These oil-based products soften the cerumen permitting easier removal from the external ear canal. Squalene appears to be well tolerated in the middle ear[3] and was not associated with otic toxicity in Mansfield's study[3].

Flushes

Irrigating solutions are used to flush out debris and any cleaning agents, such as ceruminolytics or chemical depilatories. They are also preferable in sensitive ears especially where there is ulceration and where there is mucous. A water-based flush helps break up the discharge to allow it to be removed more effectively from the ear. Generally they are administered in a gentle stream, the overflow being monitored to assess when flushed debris ceases to be present. Extreme care is needed if the tympanum is ruptured. A solution of propylene glycol and malic, benzoic, and salicylic acids, 2% or 5% acetic acid alone, or 1:3 povidone–iodine (1%) solution have been recommended if the tympanum is not intact[2,4,6]. A solution of 0.2% chlorhexidine has also been shown to be safe when instilled into the middle ear of dogs[7].

Water or sterile saline

These are the agents of choice when the integrity of the tympanum has not been established[1,7]. Given that the antimicrobial agents listed below have potential ototoxic effects, particularly in the presence of a ruptured tympanum, the justification for their use is debatable; their main indication is a broad-spectrum antimicrobial activity. However, in most cases the cleaning and irrigation procedure is a preliminary step whose function is to clean the ear canal in preparation for specific topical medication.

Chlorhexidine

A 0.2% solution of chlorhexidine acetate has a broad-spectrum antimicrobial action, may have some residual activity, and is not toxic in the presence of a ruptured tympanum in dogs, although it may exert a transient ototoxicity in cats[12,13]. An even more dilute preparation (0.0075%: 15 ml 2% solution in 4.5 litres of water) has been recommended by one author[8,11]. *Pseudomonas aeruginosa* may be resistant to chlorhexidine at this lower concentration[1].

Although concentrations of chlorhexidine diacetate over 0.013% were shown to be cytotoxic to fibroblasts *in vitro*[14], a concentration of 0.05% was not detrimental to wound healing *in vivo*[15]. However, a 0.5% solution of chlorhexidine has been shown significantly to impair granulation tissue production and wound healing[16].

On the basis of the above research a 0.05% concentration of chlorhexidine would appear to be a safe product with which to irrigate the canine external ear canal, although it might not be an ideal choice for postoperative irrigation following aural surgery. Note that *P. aeruginosa* may be resistant to chlorhexidine at a concentration of 0.05% or lower[1]. Consequently, more potent antimicrobial agents should be used if gram-negative bacterial infection is suspected.

Povidone–iodine

The bactericidal activity of povidone–iodine is related to the concentration of noncomplexed iodine in solution[17]. Concentrations of povidone–iodine greater than 0.5% are toxic to fibroblastic cultures[14], somewhat below the 1%

minimum concentration required for reliable antistaphylococcal activity[18], although comfortably above the 0.001% dilution reported to be staphylococcidal in another study[19]. However, povidone–iodine, particularly when combined with a detergent, is potentially ototoxic[20] and it is not recommended for use as a flushing agent[7].

Acetic acid

Dilute solutions of acetic acid (5% diluted 1 in 2 or 1 in 3) have been reported to be safe for use as a middle ear flushing agent[7] and several commercial preparations of 2.5% or 5% solutions are available. A recent study[18] has shown an ear cleaner containing 2% acetic acid exhibited excellent activity against *Pseudomonas* spp. A 5% solution kills staphylococci[4], although the higher concentration may be irritating.

ASSESSING THE CANAL

Cleaners should not only be selected on the type of discharge but also on the appearance of the ear canal. Cleaners of low pH and those that contain alcohol can induce further inflammation in sensitive ears (often seen in allergic animals) or ulcerated ears, often animals with gram-negative infection. Similarly, ceruminolytic agents tend to be more irritating than ceruminosolvent-based cleaners. Where an irritant cleaner is used and causes discomfort to the dog or cat it may not allow cleaning or application of ear drops to the ear on a subsequent occasion.

Some ear cleaners have been shown to have antibacterial and/or antiyeast activity in their own right. Although it is difficult to be sure which components of an ear cleaner provide it with such activity, certain components of cleaners such as chlorhexidine, povidone–iodine and acetic acid have been shown to have antipathogenic effects (see section on Flushes). Other products thought to have similar activity are ethylenediamine tetra-acetic acid tromethamine (EDTA-tris)[14–16,18,21,22], lactic acid[23,24]; isopropyl alcohol[20], parachlorometaxylenol (PCMX)[20], cleaners that contain microbial adhesion-blocking carbohydrate[25], and cleaners with a low pH[20].

EDTA-tris

EDTA binds divalent cations, enhances membrane permeability, and alters ribosome stability[14]. *P. aeruginosa* and *Staphylococcus pseudintermedius*, which are resistant to enrofloxacin and cephalexin (respectively), may be rendered sensitive by pretreatment of the external ear canal with EDTA-tris[15]. Other workers[22] have shown EDTA-tris potentiates the activity of ampicillin, chloramphenicol, oxytetracycline, and streptomycin up to fourfold. *In vitro* studies with *Pseudomonas* spp. isolated from cases of canine otitis have also demonstrated the bactericidal potential of EDTA-tris[16].

It is normally recommended that the ear canal is treated with a minimum of 2.5 ml of the EDTA-tris solution 10 minutes prior to application of antibacterial solution (such as gentamicin, cephalexin, or a gyrase inhibitor), twice daily for 7–10 days. In many countries, EDTA-tris is available commercially in an otic preparation as either an aqueous solution or as a flush combined with chlorhexidine (EDTA-tris/0.15% chlorhexidine). This latter combination has been shown to have good activity against a range of both gram-positive and gram-negative otic pathogens, the most susceptible of which were shown to be *S. pseudintermedius*, *Malassezia pachydermatis*, *Streptococcus canis*, and *Corynebacterium auricanis*[21]. The same combined solution was also shown to have good activity against *Pseudomonas* spp.[18].

Other agents with antibacterial or antiyeast activity

An ear cleaner containing 0.1% lactic acid and 2.5% salicylic acid has been shown by several studies[23, 24] to have good activity against *S. pseudintermedius*, *P. aeruginosa*, and *M. pachydermatis*. Of 31 ears from 16 dogs, 67% of animal's infection resolved within 2 weeks of twice daily application[24]. Cleaners containing microbial adhesion-blocking carbohydrates have been shown to have good antibacterial and antiyeast activity[25]. One study[20] has suggested that isopropyl alcohol and PCMX provide cleaners with antibacterial properties; these data were not supported by a larger study[18] which showed ear cleaners containing these components had inconsistent activity against bacteria. The same study[18] showed that low pH does not necessarily confer good antibacterial properties.

CLEANING PROCESS

There are three methods, not mutually exclusive, to accomplish removal of cerumen from the external ear canal[16]: mechanical removal, suction, and lavage.

Mechanical removal

This is the safest method for removing cerumen since it does not involve any risk to the tympanum or middle ear. Good visualization is imperative and if possible, both eyes should be used as this increases depth perception[16]. A wire loop, or blunt curette, is gently pulled along the lining of the canal, loosening and rolling cerumen out of the canal as it moves. After pretreatment with lubricants or ceruminolytics, there should be no tightly adherent pieces of cerumen, but if any are remaining, perhaps bound to hair shafts, they should not be subject to undue force as this may result in erosions to the epidermis.

Suction

Suction is particularly useful when cerumen is semiliquid or purulent. It is indicated for draining the middle ear[4] and is useful when the tympanum has been ruptured since there is no lavage fluid which might enter the middle ear cavity. However, there is a risk of the suction tip becoming blocked[16], and in animals the tip

is often too large to enter the middle ear[4]. Furthermore, the lack of infusion fluid can make effective cleaning difficult. The length of time involved in cleaning the equipment is also a disadvantage[4].

Irrigation

Irrigation is necessary to remove ceruminolytics or chemical depilatory compounds and it is very effective in cleaning the external ear canal[16]. Pressure irrigation is potentially hazardous as a damaged tympanum may be ruptured by powerful jets of fluid[4,16]. Curved heads on the end of the jets may help to prevent direct pressure on the tympanum[4]. The main disadvantage of many models of irrigating pump is the lack of suction, the mess they create, and the time taken to dry the dog and clean up the equipment[6]. Some models (such as the OtoPet Earigator), however, allow both irrigation and suction, in an independently adjustable manner.

Griffin[4] described using a soft rubber feeding tube attached to a syringe, which may be used alternatively to flush and aspirate fluid under direct observation through the otoscope. This method is also ideal for flushing the middle ear cavity.

Chemical depilatories

Chemical depilatory compounds have occasionally been advocated as aids in cleaning the external ear canal of dogs[12]. Given that in some dogs the external ear canal may be so hirsute that cleaning and adequate visualization is difficult, depilatory compounds would appear to be useful. Furthermore, chemical depilatory products, because of their alkalinity, might well be of value in helping to break down some of the aggregates of hair and cerumen which occur in some ears.

Most modern chemical depilatories contain thioglycolic acid or glycolate salts, presented as a cream or foam spray[13]. The depilation is accomplished by chemical disruption of disulphide bonds. The chemical effect requires a concentration of at least 2.5% and most contain thioglycolates in the range of 2.5–4%[13]. One drawback of these preparations is that thioglycolates require a very high pH (ideally about 12.5) if the chemical depilation is to occur within a few minutes[13], and as such they might be expected to have an irritant potential to dogs and cats[12]. However, one study[12] looked at the post application histopathological features of the external ear canal of dogs, and no significant evidence of inflammation was reported. Furthermore, experimental studies comparing chemical depilation with shaving found no evidence of either increased bacterial colonization or delayed wound healing[14,15].

The depilatory compound is applied via a syringe in sufficient quantity to coat the external ear canal and it is allowed to remain for 5–10 minutes before being flushed out. It has been suggested (Fadok, communication on VetDerm Listserv) that an initial test dose should be applied to the concave surface of the pinna as a few individuals may show extreme sensitivity. It is recommended that chemical depilatory compounds do not enter the middle ear.

Drying agents

Once the ear canal has been cleaned it must be dried, as residual moisture may potentiate bacterial infection. Lavage fluid may be removed by suction, or even gentle use of swabs (see above); however, where possible a drying agent should be used as a final rinse, and an alcohol-based product is recommended[1,2,6].

Most products contain isopropyl alcohol, often combined with a weak acid such as boric acid, benzoic acid, salicylic acid, or acetic acid[1,4]. High concentrations of these weak acids may be mildly irritant, particularly in inflamed ear canals and are therefore not suitable in all cases. Similarly most drying agents are ototoxic or have an unknown ototoxicity so should be used with care if the ear drum cannot be visualized[26].

HOME CLEANING

Animals with chronic and/or recurrent otitis externa benefit from regular ear cleaning which in most cases owners can perform at home, providing patient compliance is good. The most usual candidates are dogs with ceruminous otitis externa, secondary to defects in keratinization or allergy[4], and those recovered from severe bacterial infection especially where it is has been caused by multiply resistant strains of bacteria such as methicillin-resistant *Staphylococcus* or *Pseudomonas* spp. Animals with recurrent ceruminous otitis benefit from a cleaner with good ceruminolytic/ceruminosolvent activity. Many of the ceruminolytic cleaners incorporate a drying agent making the use of a second flush unnecessary. Ceruminosolvent agents often do not contain a drying agent which should therefore be employed after cleaning with a lubricant, when used on a long-term basis, to prevent colonization of the ear with bacteria or yeast. Where animals have recovered from bacterial infection, a cleaner with antiseptic qualities (e.g. containing EDTA-tris, acetic acid, chlorhexidine, or lactic acid) may be useful.

DEALING WITH PRIMARY TRIGGERS

Ectoparasites

The most important ectoparasites to affect the ears of dogs and cats are discussed in Chapter 3. In the cat, *Otodectes cynotis* accounts for up to 80% of all cases of otitis externa. Otodectic acariasis is a less common cause of otitis externa in the dog, perhaps because of the widespread use of potent systemic acaricidal spot-on medications.

Many cats develop a local hypersensitivity to *O. cynotis*[1]. These animals exhibit otitis externa characterized by variable erythema, variable pruritus, and a crumbly black-brown discharge (see Chapter 3 Aetiology and Pathogenesis of Otitis Externa). Some animals may exhibit local self-trauma, whereas others may harbour huge numbers of mites within the external ear canal and show no obvious sign of discomfort. These are easily recognized and treated. Animals exhibiting intense self-trauma with little obvious pathology are more difficult to diagnose, as are those with only one or two mites in the external ear canal: the mites are sufficient in number to cause disease but very hard to see. Problems with diagnosis may also occur in multicat households, where control may be difficult and low numbers of mites are endemic.

Combined environmental, otic, and topical (or systemic) acaricidal treatment should be carried out in these cases. Ivermectin is particularly useful as it will eliminate mites within the ear canal and any ectopic mites on the body surface. It is important that all animals in the household are treated, whether dogs or cats[2].

Other ectoparasites to affect the ears of dogs and cats include *Demodex canis* (dog), *Demodex felis* and *D. gatoi* (cat), harvest mites (*Neotrombicula autumnalis*, *Eutrombicula alfredugesi*), and ticks (*Otobius megnini*); see Chapter 3 for more details.

Ectoparasitic agents used against otic parasites

Where the ear canal contains a thick ceruminous discharge, prior cleaning of the ear with a ceruminolytic may be beneficial to remove discharge and facilitate the penetration of the topical ectoparasiticide. Many different commercial otic preparations are licensed for the therapy of otic ectoparasites; the reader is referred to individual product data sheets for further details.

Monosulfiram (tetraethylthiuran monosulphide)

Indication: *Otodectes cynotis*.

Sulphur has been used for centuries as a scabicide and monosulfiram emulsion has a long history as a topical acaricide[3]. However, it is rarely used in human dermatology as it cross-reacts with alcohol abuse treatments[4]. Monosulfiram also has a fungicidal effect and a 5 mg/ml solution is active against malassezial yeast[5].

Thiabendazole (2-(thiazol-4-yl) benzimidazole)

Indications: *Malassezia pachydermatis, Aspergillus* spp., *O. cynotis*, ticks, feline otodemodicosis.

Thiabendazole is an antifungal agent with acaricidal properties[6]. Thiabendazole kills all stages of the mite life cycle[7] and is thus preferred to pyrethrins and rotenone, for example, which have no activity against eggs. Thiabendazole is useful against malassezial yeast and otodectic mites[7,8] and its lack of toxicity, in standard doses, has made it a popular ingredient in otic polypharmaceutical preparations. A topical otic preparation containing thiabendazole, neomycin, and dexamethasone has also been reported to be curative against *O. megnini* ticks[9]. Thiabendazole is also effective in the treatment of feline otodemodicosis[7].

Pyrethrin, pyrethroids, carbamates, and rotenone

Indications: *O. cynotis, N. autumnalis, E. alfredurgesi*, tick infestation.

These are relatively broad-spectrum insecticides and acaricides. Pyrethrins (natural derivatives of Chrysanthemum such as cinerariaefolium), pyrethroids (synthetic analogues), and rotenone are characterized by quick knock-down and poor persistence. They are thus commonly used in over-the-counter antiparasitic preparations for puppies and kittens. These agents all have similar spectra of activity and a low toxicity potential, although if cats are treated with products marketed for dogs, toxic side-effects may be seen[10,11]. None of these agents kill the eggs of ear mites and thus repeated treatment is necessary.

Ivermectin

Indications: *Demodex* spp., *O. cynotis, Sarcoptes scabiei, Notoedres cati, N. autumnalis*, ticks, *Linognathus setosus*.

Ivermectin is effective against demodectic and sarcoptic mange in dogs, at doses of 0.3 mg/kg body weight[12]. It is given on four occasions at 7-day intervals for scabies, and once daily until remission is achieved for demodicosis[13]. Ivermectin has been advocated for otodectic mange in cats[13,14] at a dose of 0.2–0.3 mg/kg. Two injections at 10–14 day intervals are curative. Although ivermectin may be administered topically, orally, or by injection, the topical route is least effective[14]. Subcutaneous injections must only be given using the propylene glycol-based presentation[15]. For oral dosing, particularly long-term treatment, it may be more appropriate to use the water-based presentation marketed for oral administration to the horse, although it may prove difficult to measure the exact dose. This will obviate any risk of propylene-glycol toxicity which, although rare, may be noted occasionally (bradycardia and central nervous system and respiratory depression).

Ivermectin should be highly effective against other mites affecting cats and dogs[13]. It has some activity against the sucking louse of dogs (*L. setosus*) and some activity against ticks; it inhibits feeding and the ticks fall off only partially engorged.

Certain breeds of dog are susceptible to side-effects when given ivermectin, and great care is warranted when considering its use. Informed, preferably signed, consent may be necessary in some circumstances. Ivermectin toxicity is related to central nervous system effects caused by ivermectin-enhanced gamma-amino butyric acid (GABA) activity[15]. In most canine breeds acute toxicity is seen when a dose in excess of 2.5 mg/kg is given. In cats the maximum dose above which signs of acute toxicity are seen is 0.75 mg/kg orally. Chronic toxicity begins to be noted with doses in excess of 1 mg/kg in dogs and 0.5 mg/kg in cats[15]. There appears to be minimal risk of teratogenic effects following administration of ivermectin to pregnant bitches[15]. Signs of ivermectin toxicity include mydriasis, depression, tremors, ataxia, stupor, emesis, coma, and death[15–17]. However, certain breeds of dogs exhibit an idiosyncratic sensitivity to ivermectin, developing side-effects at doses as low as 0.1 mg/kg. Collies, Old English Sheepdogs, and Shetland Sheepdogs are particularly susceptible[15].

Ivermectin dosages over 0.05 mg/kg will kill *Dirofilaria immitis* larvae. Therefore, in heartworm-endemic areas dogs should be tested for heartworm before receiving ivermectin in acaricidal dosages[15].

Many dogs with ivermectin toxicity will recover, particularly if recognized early and treated adequately. The provision of adequate nursing care is critical[16] and treatment is based on antishock doses of glucocorticoids and intravenous fluids[16,17]. Specific agents that may antagonize ivermectin include picrotoxin and physostigmine. Clinicians are unlikely to be able to obtain these agents easily or quickly.

The inability to predict with any confidence if an individual dog will exhibit ivermectin toxicity is one of the main problems facing clinicians[16]. A modified dosing schedule has been proposed which provides for a gradually increasing dose, allowing the opportunity to observe the dogs closely for toxic signs[12]. Prompt intervention (and at the subcritical dose stage) increases the chances of recovery from ivermectin toxicity. The modified dosing scheme is as follows[12]:

- Day 1 – 0.05 mg/kg
- Day 2 – 0.1 mg/kg
- Day 3 – 0.15 mg/kg
- Day 4 – 0.2 mg/kg
- Day 5 – 0.3 mg/kg

Amitraz

Indications: *Demodex* spp., *S. scabiei*, ticks.

Amitraz is a monoamine oxidase inhibitor presented in an organic vehicle. Although serious side-effects are rare, owners may report transient lethargy and hypothermia post dipping[18,19]. Bradycardia, hypertension, and hyperglycaemia may be seen in some animals[18,20]. Problems are most serious in very small dogs where the hypothermia may be severe. The drug is contraindicated in Chihuahuas, for example. Precautions must be taken to prevent operator exposure[19] and the dipping should be performed in a well-ventilated room. The person carrying out the dipping should wear gloves and waterproof protective clothing. Recommended treatment of canine otodemodicosis is 1 ml of 19.9% amitraz solution in 30 ml mineral oil, or 2 ml 5% solution in 20 ml mineral oil[7,21,22].

Amitraz is also licensed (in the UK) against scabies, at a dilution of 0.025% (25 ml 5% solution in 5 litres of water).

Amitraz preparations are useful as a tick repellent[23] and in some countries the chemical is marketed as an amitraz-impregnated collar for this purpose. Accidental ingestion of amitraz-impregnated collars may prove fatal to dogs and prompt treatment is necessary. Atipamezole (50 µg/kg i/m) should be followed by oral yohimbine (0.1 mg/kg) every 6 hours as needed[20].

Fipronil

Indications: *Spilopsyllus cuniculi*, *O. cynotis*, *S. scabies*, *N. autumnalis*, ticks, lice.

Fipronil is primarily marketed as a flea control product and as such it will be effective against *S. cuniculi*. Although presented in both spray and spot-on formulations, the spray formulation is preferred for the treatment of otic parasites since effective local concentrations on both hair and skin surfaces may be achieved rapidly. Fipronil has also been used off license as a topical otic application. Fipronil is also effective against lice[24].

Fipronil has been demonstrated under field conditions to prevent infestation with trombiculid mites and ticks[25,26]. The spray formulation of fipronil is preferred for this indication. Fipronil spray has also proven effective against scabies[27] and it may be particularly useful when clinicians are faced with scabies in very young puppies, where other topical treatments are inadvisable.

Selamectin

Indications: *S. scabiei*, *O.cynotis*, possibly *S. cuniculi*, lice.

Selamectin is a novel avermectin with considerable advantages over ivermectin:

- It is safe in ivermectin-sensitive Collies[28].
- It is effective against fleas, roundworms, hookworms, and heartworm[29,30] in addition to *O. cynotis* and *S. scabiei*.
- It is applied topically.

Selamectin must not be given to animals of less than 6 weeks of age and it must be applied topically to the back of the neck, even for the treatment of *O. cynotis*.

Allergic otitis
Canine otitis externa associated with hypersensitivity

In the dog more than 75% of cases of otitis externa are caused by allergy[31,32]. The most common hypersensitivity to affect the canine ear is atopy, although food intolerance and contact allergy/irritancy may also cause otitis externa. In the acute stages of allergy the canal responds to inflammation with erythema, oedema, and hyperplasia, often with minimal microbial multiplication. When microbial proliferation occurs it is usually staphylococcal and malassezial in nature, rather than gram negative.

On the first presentation of otitis externa investigation of a primary trigger is unjustified, but where disease is recurrent it is essential to prevent progression to chronic change. On the first occasion, damage to the tympanic membrane and concurrent otitis media is unlikely but the tympanum should still be assessed. Basic steps on the first presentation should include:

- Identification of secondary infection by cytology and topical therapy of secondary malassezial and bacterial multiplication.

- Apply topical otic glucocorticoids to suppress inflammation, reduce epithelial hyperproliferation, and minimize fibrosis. The potency of the glucocorticoids should depend on the degree of erythema and hyperplasia in the canal. Where mild to moderate change is present prednisolone may be suitable; where there is more severe inflammation more potent topical drugs such as betamethasone, dexamethasone, hydrocortisone aceponate, or mometasone may be more suitable.
- Maintain remission with regular application of otic cleansers, antimicrobial ointments, and occasional otic glucocorticoid preparations.
- Caution owners of breeds in which atopy is well recognized about allergic otitis and the importance of prompt attention if recurrence occurs.

Application of topical glucocorticoids to these ear canals (and to the concave aspect of the pinnae) can produce a spectacular reduction in the degree of inflammation and otic stenosis which is present, often obviating the requirement for surgery. However, regular use of potent glucocorticoids, even in otic preparations, can induce iatrogenic hyper-adreno-corticism[1]. Therefore, although a potent fluorinated steroid may initially be indicated, the clinician should switch to a minimally potent agent such as prednisolone, prednisone, or hydrocortisone for maintenance.

Where animals present with recurrent allergic otitis then investigation is essential. All cases should be food trialled using a home cooked exclusion diet or a proprietary hydrolyzed diet. *In vitro* or *in vivo* allergy testing (for environmental allergens NOT foods allergens) may also be useful especially where inflammation and pruritus is present on other areas of the body, especially the muzzle and periocular areas. This gives the clinician the opportunity to use allergen specific therapy immunotherapy as part of the therapeutic regime to control both skin disease and the otitis externa.

Allergic contact dermatitis to otic medications has been reported, most commonly to neomycin and propylene glycol. Whether the reaction to propylene glycol is a true allergic reaction and not simply an irritant dermatitis is not clear. An allergic contact reaction should be suspected when the application of topical medication causes an increase in discomfort or pain. Treatment should consist of removal of all topical medication and the institution of a 5–7-day course of prednisolone at a dose of 1 mg/kg by mouth once daily. Subsequent topical therapy may be reintroduced with care, but a detailed knowledge of the composition of each product should be sought before use.

Feline otitis associated with hypersensitivity

Although atopy is a very common cause of otitis externa in dogs, it appears to be much less so in cats, perhaps due to differences in anatomy, such as a relatively wide canal, lack of hair within the canal, and an upright pinna[8]. There may also be differences in the cerumen which make microbial overgrowth less likely, even in the face of chronic inflammation. Intradermal skin testing is more difficult to perform in the cat compared to dogs, and many clinicians will make a provisional diagnosis of atopy on the basis of ruling out all other potential diagnoses. Dietary intolerance (food allergy) is also rare in the cat. However, pinnal erythema and otitis externa may be associated with intolerance to dietary components[33]. Perhaps more commonly, there is facial and head pruritus with the pinnae and periaural areas being affected, rather than the external ear canals[33–35]. The most common allergens in proven cases of feline dietary intolerance are beef, milk, and fish[36]. Diagnosis is based

on a resolution of the clinical signs while an exclusion diet is fed. A period of 3–16 weeks may elapse before complete recovery is noted. Allergic contact dermatitis is extraordinarily rare in cats. However, allergic contact dermatitis to topical neomycin is recognized by some clinicians. Certainly, the diagnosis should be considered in all cases of refractory otitis externa.

Otitis externa associated with a defect in keratinization

Ceruminous otitis externa is not always complicated by infection, but chronic cases usually are. In particular there is a tendency for gram-negative bacteria to proliferate early in the course of the disease and this must be identified and treated. Furthermore, there may be concurrent otitis media and this must be ruled in or ruled out before long-term measures are instituted:

- Keep the external ear canal and the surrounding area as clean as possible. Pluck hair regularly out of the external ear canal, and keep the concave aspect of the proximal pinna and surrounding area clipped short. Local shampooing may be helpful in keeping greasy scale to a minimum; use a degreasing, keratolytic, or keratoplastic product such as benzyl peroxide or one of the tar/sulphur/salicylic acid combination products.
- Regular use of an acetic acid-based aqueous cleanser (2.5% or 5% concentration) will help to keep the otic pH acid and suppress gram-negative overgrowth. Commercial products may be used, as may equal quantities of white vinegar and water, or alcohol[2,3].
- Regular use of ear cleansers which loosen cerumen and inhibit microbial growth may help to prevent accumulation of such debris and prevent relapse into overt otitis externa.

- Occasional, sometimes more frequent, use of cleansers such as carbamide peroxide, dioctyl sodium sulfosuccinate, or squalene will help to flush out accumulations of ceruminous debris, although a drying agent, such as one based on isopropyl alcohol, should be used after these products[37].
- Otic polypharmaceutical preparations with combinations of glucocorticoids and antimicrobial agents, based on bacterial culture and sensitivity, may be indicated if the measures outlined above fail to prevent otitis externa developing.

Proliferative otitis

This is a rare condition, with an almost pathognomonic presentation, that can affect both kittens and adult cats[38]. The condition typically presents as a bilateral, occasionally malodorous, chronic otitis externa. Large, dark red, brownish, almost vegetative, proliferative plaques with necrotic surfaces can be seen, at the base of the pinnae and the upper portions of the vertical ear canal (Figure 5.1). The tissue and exudates may occlude the ear canal. Removal of the rather loosely adherent overlying proliferative tissue results in ulceration and erosions to the underlying tissue. Histopathological examination reveals prominent hyperkeratosis and apoptopic keratinocytes, presumably reflecting an immune-mediated process[39]

Topical tacrolimus ointment twice daily is very effective: some cases appear to go into full time remission, others require maintenance therapy.

DEALING WITH SECONDARY CAUSES

Topical versus systemic therapy

> ### KEY POINTS
>
> - Topical therapy is the key to successful resolution of otitis externa which is essentially a surface infection.
> - Although controversial it is unlikely, except possibly in situations where the canal is eroded or ulcerated, that systemic drugs will reach therapeutic concentrations within the discharge within the canal.
> - It is essential to use adequate volumes of both cleaning solution and topical medication to ensure it penetrates the discharge.
> - In the initial stages of therapy, topical medication can be selected empirically based on cytological examination of the discharge, examination of the canal, and the presence or absence of the tympanic membrane.

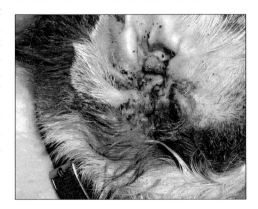

Fig. 5.1 Almost pathognomic signs of feline proliferative otitis: vegetative plaques with surface necrosis. (Courtesy of Dr. Brenda Stevens, College of Veterinary Medicine, North Carolina State University, Raleigh.)

Malassezial yeast and otitis externa

KEY POINTS

- Most commonly yeast otitis externa in the dog is caused by *M. pachydermatis* and in the cat by *M. pachydermatis* and *M. sympodialis*[40].
- Malassezial yeast is a common secondary infection in cases of acute allergy and in keratinization disorders.
- Cytology is the best method to identify yeast and is more specific than culture.
- Antifungal therapy is usually curative but where recurrence occurs, an underlying primary cause should be sought.

Clinical signs

Malassezial otitis is usually bilateral and pruritic rather than painful. Damage to the tympanic membrane in acute disease is uncommon. Underlying primary causes include allergy, particularly atopy, and both primary and secondary keratinization disorders. In the dog, the most common secondary disorder of keratinization is endocrine disease in the form of hypothyroidism and hyper-adrenocorticism. In the cat, malassezial infection can be seen secondary to systemic disease, such as pancreatic or hepatic disease, and is commonly associated with hyperthyroidism. Ears with ceruminous otitis, especially where there is epidermal hyperplasia with partial occlusion of the canal, are predisposed to developing yeast infection.

Treatment

Before application of a topical antifungal drug it is important that the ear is cleaned adequately. Ceruminolytic / ceruminosolvent cleaners are best employed to remove thick ceruminous discharge before application of otic drops (see Chapter 4 Ear Cleaning). Many different antifungal drugs are available in a wide range of commercial otic preparations to treat malassezial otitis; most are combined with an antibiotic and a glucocorticoid. Where there is yeast infection coupled with chronic change, especially where there is narrowing of the canal with glandular hyperplasia, then it is advantageous if the antifungal drug is combined with a potent topical glucocorticoid such as betamethasone, dexamethasone, mometasone, or hydro-cortisone aceponate. Once chronic change has been reversed, therapy should be switched to a less potent glucocorticoid such as prednisolone.

Polyenes

Nystatin is a polyene antifungal that works by binding to sterols in the fungal cell membrane, changing permeability and leading to fungal death by osmotic destruction. Nystatin has activity against both *Candida* spp. and *M. pachydermatis*. In European countries it is available as a commercial drop combined with fusidic acid, framycetin, and prednisolone.

Azoles

The azole antifungal drugs all disrupt the biosynthesis of the fungal cell wall ergosterol by inhibition of P450 enzyme. Topical azole is available as imidazoles (clotrimazole, miconazole, ketoconazole) and as triazoles (itraconazole, posa-conazole). All of the azole drugs have excellent *in vitro* activity against *Malassezia* spp. A number of studies have rated the potency of the azoles differently. A study[41] suggested itraconazole was the most potent of the drugs followed by ketoconazole, miconazole, and clotrima-zole. A more recent *in vitro* study[42] showed that ketoconazole, itraconazole, and ter-binafine were equally potent. Only com-mercial studies have compared the second generation triazole posaconazole with the imidazole clotrimazole, suggesting posaconazole is at least 10 times more potent. Oral ketoconazole or itraconazole has been described as useful systemic therapy for malassezial otitis in dogs, whereas itraconazole is preferred in cats[43].

Allylamines

Allylamines disrupt ergosterol biosynthesis and therefore prevent cell wall formation by inhibition of the enzyme squalene epoxidase. Terbinafine is the most widely available antifungal in this class; it has good activity against malassezial species. There are no veterinary topical preparations available, although a 1% terbinafine cream has been used as an otic preparation in dogs off license.

Gram-positive otitis externa

KEY POINTS

- Gram-positive otitis externa in the dog is most commonly caused by coagulase positive *Staphylococcus pseudintermedius*.
- Staphylococcal infection is a common secondary infection in cases of allergy in dogs and cats; it can occur in mixed growth with *Streptococcus* spp. and *M. pachydermatis*.
- Both *Staphylococcus* and *Streptococcus* spp. appear as cocci on cytology.
- Bacterial culture and sensitivity testing should be undertaken when infection has failed to respond to rational therapy, in which case methicillin-resistant *Staphylococcus aureus* (MRSA) or methicillin-resistant *S. pseudintermedius* may be present.

Clinical signs

Gram-positive otitis externa usually produces mildly pruritic, unilateral or bilateral otitis with a yellow brown purulent discharge. Allergy is the most common underlying primary cause of infection and the affected ear canal is usually sensitive, erythematous, and hyperplastic; changes often involve the medial aspect of the pinna in addition to the canal. In chronic disease, ongoing or recurrent infection can lead to otitis media. Chronic topical and systemic antibiotic usage can predispose to the development of multiply resistant isolates of both methicillin-resistant *Staphylococcus pseudintermedius*, MRSA, and *Enterococcus faecalis*.

Treatment

Therapy should be prescribed where possible with topical drugs with a narrow spectrum of activity. Drugs such as fluoroquinolones, carboxypenicillins, and third generation cephalosporins should be reserved where possible for gram-negative infections involving *Pseudomonas* spp., and should be prescribed on the basis of culture and sensitivity. Drugs such as aminoglycosides are inactive in purulent material and, therefore, thorough cleaning of the ear should be performed using an antiseptic flush (see Chapter 4 Ear Cleaning) before application of antibacterial otic drops. Where infection occurs in chronically damaged ears, for example where there is narrowing of the canal, topical antibiotics are best combined with a potent topical glucocorticoid (see chronic change in antifungal therapy above). In allergic otitis where maintenance therapy with topical glucocorticoids is useful, otic drops may be continued to be used. However, although long-term use of topical steroids may be beneficial, chronic topical antibiotic usage should be avoided. This is often impossible when prescription otic preparations contain an antibiotic and a glucocorticoid. In such cases off-licensed usage of an antiseptic cleaner is used by the author combined with a glucocorticoid such as injectable dexamethasone.

Fusidic acid

Fusidic acid is a narrow spectrum bacteriostatic antimicrobial. Its spectrum is limited to gram-positive cocci and therefore constitutes a good first-line empirical choice for staphylococcal infection.

Aminoglycosides

Aminoglycosides are common components of topical otic preparations. This group contains among others, amikacin, framycetin, gentamicin, neomycin, and tobramycin. Amikacin and tobramycin should, in the author's opinion, be reserved for use against gram-negative bacteria and will be discussed in that section.

Framycetin

Framycetin is a broad spectrum bactericidal aminoglycoside with good activity against *Staphylococcus* spp. as well as many different gram-negative organisms including *Pseudomonas* spp. It is a good first-line choice for topical therapy when cocci are identified on cytology. It is available in Europe as part of a commercial veterinary otic medication.

Neomycin

Neomycin has the lowest potency of all the aminoglycosides. It has limited activity against gram-negative bacteria, such as *Pseudomonas* spp., but good activity against gram-positive cocci. Neomycin is a good first-line drug for acute bacterial otitis when cocci predominate cytologically[44]. Neomycin is one of the most commonly implicated topical agents for contact hypersensitivity/irritancy in the dog.

Gentamicin

Gentamicin has excellent activity against gram-positive cocci and some activity against gram-negative bacteria[45]. A wide range of veterinary commercial products are available containing gentamicin combined with a range of different antifungal drugs and glucocorticoids. Selection of product is often determined by the strength of the glucocorticoids when the antibiotic in products is the same. Despite anecdotal concern over the ototoxic potential of gentamicin, a study in dogs designed to stimulate clinical exposure via a ruptured tympanic membrane failed to document any toxicity[46]. Where reactions to topical gentamicin preparations have been recorded, it may therefore have been the vehicle that produced side-effects rather than the antibiotic. Gentamicin can be used mixed with ethylenediamine tetra-acetic acid tromethamine (EDTA-tris) as an off-license formulation when the tympanum is damaged[47]:

- 4×2 ml vials of 40 mg/ml can be added to 118 ml of EDTA-tris and used effectively to treat both gram-positive and gram-negative infections.

Gram-negative otitis externa

KEY POINTS

- Gram-negative otitis externa is usually acute in onset, suppurative, and painful[48].
- Bathing, grooming, and foreign bodies are the most common conditions associated with acute gram-negative otitis externa.
- Bacterial culture and sensitivity testing is mandatory as multiple-resistant strains may be recovered.
- 2% or 2.5% acetic acid may be used for treatment on an empirical basis pending laboratory results.

Clinical signs

Most cases of gram-negative otitis externa are acute in onset, unilateral, painful rather than pruritic, suppurative, and ulcerated[49]. The most common causes in one survey of 550 dogs with otitis externa were otic foreign body, grooming, and bathing, rather than underlying disease[39]. This finding was supported in another large study (of 752 dogs with otitis externa) in which underlying disease was not a feature of gram-negative otitis in dogs[50].

Otic inflammation, an increase in humidity, and a rise in pH within the external ear canal appear to be necessary for *Pseudomonas* spp. to establish[48]; inflammation *per se* is not sufficient in the normal external ear canal. However, predisposing factors, such as hirsute ear canals, narrow ear canals, and pendulous pinnae, may make the external ear canal more susceptible to gram-negative infection. Hence, Cocker Spaniels are predisposed[51]. Gram-negative infections of the external ear canal appear to be more common in tropical climates, possibly because of increased temperature and increased humidity in the environment affecting, or potentiating, alteration in the otic microclimate.

Treatment

Note that, to date, there have been no blinded studies into the optimum treatment protocol for pseudomonal otitis[50], meaning that the clinicians have only limited data on which to make a therapeutic decision; every case must be taken on merit and based on culture and sensitivity.

The aims of therapy in pseudomonal otitis should be to:
- Clean the ear thoroughly to remove exudate which is usually mucopurulent.
- Kill, or remove, the pseudomonal bacteria
- Decrease inflammation and further production of exudates.
- Reverse chronic changes in the ear and create an environment which is hostile to pseudomonal bacteria to prevent recolonization (see section on therapy of chronic change later in this chapter).

Note: due to the severe ulcerative painful changes that typically occur within the ear canal in these infections, the initial flushing of the ear is best undertaken in an anaesthetized animal which should have an endotracheal tube placed with the cuff inflated.

Cleaning the ear

Where there is a ceruminous discharge then a ceruminolytic, such as carbamide peroxide or dioctyl sodium sulphosuccinate, or a ceruminosolvent, such as squalene, can be used to clean the ears. Where the tympanum cannot be seen or is damaged, squalene is the safest option. More often the discharge is mucopurulent and water is the best initial flush. Large volumes of sterile water or isotonic saline may be used to break up the thick tenacious mucous.

Killing the Pseudomonas (1): disinfectant flushes

Although antibiotics can be used to kill *Pseudomonas* spp. and are important in ongoing therapy, topical antiseptics are beneficial after an initial water flush. The authors favour a double flush in the form of a 5 minute acid soak followed by a second 5 minute potentiating disinfectant flush:
- The first flush is with an acid-based solution such as acetic, boric, citric, or lactic acid. Vinegar diluted 50:50 with sterile water provides an acetic acid solution of 2.5% which is an excellent flush with good activity against pseudomonal bacteria. Acetic acid is the author's preferred flush especially when the ear drum is ruptured. A 2% acetic acid flush is available as a commercial otic cleaning solution in many countries.
- After an acid flush a second topical disinfectant can be used. This may be an alcohol, aluminium hydroxide, chlorhexidine (0.2% or less) or EDTA-tris. *In vitro* studies with *Pseudomonas* spp. isolated from cases of canine otitis have also demonstrated the bactericidal potential of EDTA-tris[51].

The authors favour a combination of chlorhexidine 0.15% with EDTA-tris as a second flush. The two components of this solution, which is available as a commercial flush, have been shown to have synergistic antibacterial effects[52]. In addition, EDTA-tris has been shown to have the ability to potentiate a range of antibiotics.

EDTA binds divalent cations, enhances membrane permeability, and alters ribosome stability[53]. *P. aeruginosa* and *S. intermedius*, which are resistant to enrofloxacin and cephalexin (respectively), may be rendered sensitive by pretreatment of the external ear canal with EDTA-tris[54].

Decreasing the inflammation

Inflammation within the canal can be reduced using both topical and systemic glucocorticoids. Potent topical glucocorticoids that are useful are otic preparations containing mometasone, dexamethasone, or betamethasone. Where the ear drum is damaged the safest topical steroid is off-license usage of dexamethasone sodium phosphate (2 mg/ml) which can be diluted 50:50 with water or sterile saline and instilled into the ear. Once the flushing procedure has been completed 0.25–0.5 ml of glucocorticoid solution can be instilled into the ear. An intravenous anti-inflammatory injection of an appropriate dexamethasone solution can be given before waking the animal up.

Killing the Pseudomonas (2): antibiotics

Initial therapy of the pseudomonal infection can be undertaken with a range of drugs. Silver sulfadiazine, continued use of acetic acid or topical polymyxin, aminoglycosides (framycetin, gentamicin), or fluoroquinolones (enrofloxacin, marbofloxacin, ciprofloxacin, orbifloxacin) are all suitable as empirical first-line therapy after cytology has identified the presence of rods on cytology, pending culture and sensitivity. Other drugs, such as amikacin and tobramycin, may be used second line if these drugs are found to be unsuitable. Third-line drugs, such as carboxypenicillins (carbenicillin, ticarcillin), third generation cephalosporins (ceftazidime), and imipenem, are rarely if ever indicated and should only be used when all other options have been exhausted.

Silver sulfadiazine

Silver sulfadiazine has broad spectrum antibacterial activity especially against *P. aeruginosa* but also has activity against *Staphylococcus* spp. 1% silver sulfadiazine cream applied daily for 10 days is effective but, being rather viscous in nature, it is hard to apply to the depths of the external ear canal[55]. However, dilutions of the cream with water, to a concentration as low as 1/100, will exceed the minimum inhibitory concentration (MIC) for *P. aeruginosa* and are fluid enough to penetrate the depths of the ear canal[56]. A 0.1% solution may be prepared by mixing 1.5 ml silver sulfadiazine cream into 13.5 ml water or saline[57]. This may be instilled into the ear canal twice daily. The ototoxicity of silver sulfadiazine is reported to be low[44,58]. It has though been reported to produce signs of systemic toxicity when absorbed through burn wounds in man[59] so caution should be used when applied to the ears of dogs with extensive ulceration.

Fluoroquinolone antibacterial agents

Fluoroquinolones are bactericidal antibiotics with good activity against a wide range of bacteria, especially gram-negative bacilli and gram-positive cocci (including *Staphylococcus* spp. but with variable activity against *Streptococcus* spp.)[44]. Enrofloxacin, marbofloxacin, and ciprofloxacin are highly effective against *P. aeruginosa* and *Proteus* spp.[60,61]. A topical enrofloxacin-based otic drop is available in the USA, and a specific otic preparation containing marbofloxacin, clotrimazole, and dexamethasone is available in some countries. There is evidence (manufacturer's internal data) that adjunctive treatment with systemic administration may enhance the 'time to cure interval'. In those countries where a specific fluoroquinolone-based otic preparation is not available or where the tympanum is ruptured and such products are not deemed safe, off-license usage of injectable fluoroquinolones has been employed as topical therapy. These can be used mixed with sterile water or combined with an ear cleaning solution, especially EDTA-tris which has been shown to potentiate fluoroquinolone activity. Care should be taken to ensure that the external ear canal is cleaned and thoroughly dried before instilling topical fluoroquinolones since they are inactivated in an acidic environment[54,62]. Many different dilutions of antibiotic have been suggested by different authors. A dilution of the injectable enrofloxacin solution (20 mg/ml) at the rate of 1:6 in water or isotonic saline has been recommended as being efficacious when instilled directly into the external ear canal[54]. Other dilutions include a 1:3 dilution of 2% enrofloxacin or 1% marbofloxacin injectable solution mixed with EDTA-tris[63]. Enrofloxacin made up to a concentration of 0.9% can be mixed with: 1) sterile water; 2) an EDTA-tris cleaner with and without 0.15% chlorhexidine; and 3) with a salicylic acid (0.1%) and parachlorometaxlenol (0.1%) based cleaner with either lactic acid (2.5%) or EDTA (0.5%), and maintains good chemical stability and antibacterial activity for up to 28 days[64].

Amikacin and tobramycin

Amikacin and tobramycin are both aminoglycoside antibiotics with a good activity against *P. aeruginosa*. Amikacin is not available as a commercial otic preparation but the injectable solution can be used as an off-licensed product diluted to a concentration of 30–50 mg/ml in sterile saline or EDTA-tris[47]. Tobramycin as an injectable solution may be mixed with sterile saline or EDTA-tris to a concentration of 8 mg/ml[47]. The long-term

stability of these products is unknown. Both amikacin and tobramycin are potentially ototoxic and should be used with care if the ear drum is damaged.

Other antibacterial agents

Imipenem and carbenicillin are both active against *P. aeruginosa*, although imipenem has met with resistance problems because of its widespread use in the human field[65]. Topically applied ticarcillin, in conjunction with prednisolone (1–2 mg/kg p/o q12 h) and an acetic acid-based topical otic cleanser, has been reported to be effective[66]. If the tympanum is ruptured, the ticarcillin is administered three times daily intravenously until healing is observed[65]. The topical solution is made by mixing a 6 g vial of ticarcillin powder with 12 ml of sterile water[66]. This may be divided into 2 ml aliquots and frozen, where it will remain stable for up to 3 months. The vials are thawed and mixed with 40 ml saline, each again being divided into aliquots, this time of about 10 ml. These are given to the client to freeze at home. When required they are thawed for use, the surplus being kept in the refrigerator for up to 7 days.

Use of ear wicks in the therapy of otitis externa

Ear wicks are made of polyvinyl alcohol (PVA) which forms a hard, compact structure. Dry wicks can be cut and shaped before being inserted into the external ear canal (Figure 5.2). Once positioned in the ear (Figure 5.3), the wick can be soaked in any aqueous solution allowing the sponge to expand in a controlled manner to fill the contours of the ear canal (Figure 5.4). In the author's experience they are well tolerated providing they are cut, if necessary, to an appropriate size and positioned correctly. In small dogs and cats, overly long wicks can be felt when the animals articulate their temperomandibular joint, which can lead to some discomfort on opening their jaws.

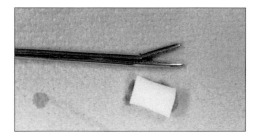

Fig. 5.2 Earwick cut to size and ready to insert into the external ear canal.

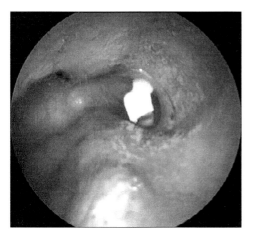

Fig. 5.3 Earwick placed into the external ear canal.

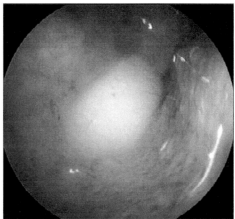

Fig. 5.4 Earwick filling the ear canal after absorbing the medicants.

Wicks can be used successfully in all but the giant dogs. In normal ears of such breeds the canals are too wide so that even when the wick is expanded they do not fill the whole canal. They can though be used to treat stenotic ear canal in these breeds. The sponge has a porous interconnected structure which gives it great tensile strength, so that it will not disintegrate or tear while *in situ* or when it is grasped to be removed. The fine pores facilitate minimal tissue adhesion providing it remains soaked. Effective cleaning of the canal is critical when wicks are used. If the canal is not adequately flushed then the wick will act as a cork to 'bottle up' infection which can then predispose to the development of otitis media. The principal uses of ear wicks in veterinary medicine are for:

- Treatment of bacterial/yeast otitis externa.
- Reduction of hyperplasia/stenosis of the external ear canal (see section later on chronic change).
- Postoperative packing after nonablative surgery.

Ear wicks can be used to treat otitis externa in cases where the dog will not tolerate or the owner is unable to apply otic drops. The wicks can be used in combination with any aqueous solution especially water-based solutions of antibiotic. Successful therapy involves several steps and is best accomplished on an anaesthetized animal:

1 Assessment of the ear canal and tympanic membrane.
2 Assessment of the otic discharge with cytology +/– culture.
3 Thorough cleaning of the canal.
4 Selection of soak solution and placement of wick.
5 Postflushing glucocorticoid administration.

1 **Assessment of the ear canal and tympanic membrane** is important to establish if the disease is confined to the external ear canal. Where the ear drum is damaged and otitis media is present therapy may be tailored to suit this (see Chapter 6 Otitis Media).
2 **Assessment of the otic discharge with cytology** +/– **culture** is essential to decide on the most appropriate drug to apply to the wick. Where cocci or yeast are present culture is not generally necessary unless the bacterial infection has already failed to respond to conventional therapy or MRSA is suspected. When rods are identified culture should be performed.
3 **Thorough cleaning of the canal** is an important step in therapy. Careful selection of an appropriate cleaning solution is essential (see Chapter 4 Ear Cleaning). The ear canal should be cleaned and ideally should then be soaked in a disinfectant solution, e.g. acetic acid, chlorhexidine/EDTA-tris, or lactic acid prior to placement of the wick.

4 **Selection of soak solution and placement of the wick**; an unsoaked wick should be placed deep in the vertical canal, extending into the horizontal canal where possible. Once positioned, the wick should be soaked. A wick will normally absorb approximately 2 ml of aqueous solution, which should be gently syringed into the ear canal. After soaking, the wick should be left *in situ* for a few minutes before being rechecked. At this stage a further 0.5 ml of fluid can be applied if necessary. The wick is adequately soaked when a small amount of fluid is seen to be pooled on the top of it. Where bacteria have been identified, by cytology, the wick may be soaked in an aqueous solution of antibiotic such as injectable solutions of fluoroquinolones (enrofloxacin, marbofloxacin), trimethoprim sulfadiazine, or aminoglycosides (gentamicin). Where indicated by sensitivity, and where other drugs have been shown to be ineffective, other aminoglycosides (amikacin, tobramycin) and carboxypenicillins (ticarcillin) may be appropriate. Where yeast is identified on cytology, enilconazole diluted 1:5 with sterile water may be used to infuse the wicks.
5 **Postflushing glucocorticoid administration**; flushing can cause irritation of the lining of the external ear canal which can lead to head shaking during the postoperative period. If the dog shakes it's head then it is possible the wick may be lost. Therefore, unless contraindicated, an intravenous bolus of dexamethasone at an anti-inflammatory dose should be administered before recovering the animal.

The animal should be discharged and the owner supplied with a small quantity (2–3 ml) of soak solution to add to the ear after 3–5 days, to ensure that the wick stays hydrated. If this is not possible the patient should revisit the surgery for a nurse to administer the additional soak solution. The dog may also be sent home with a 7–10-day course of prednisolone at a dose of 0.5–1 mg/kg to provide anti-inflammatory benefits.

Reassessment should be undertaken at 7–10 days. The dog will need to be anaesthetized again at this stage. The wick can be easily removed if it is well soaked. Approximately 2–3 ml of sterile water should be syringed into the ear to ensure adequate hydration of the wick before attempting removal. It may then be grasped with a pair of forceps and gently removed. Cytology can now be repeated, the ear reflushed and, if necessary, a further wick applied. Often at this juncture the ear is more comfortable and the owner can then administer drops. Cytology may reveal that the infection has cleared.

Liquid bandages, ear packs, and other 'stay in place' otics

In an effort to ensure constant concentrations of antibacterial agents, and with a nod to the logistic implications for busy owners with recalcitrant pets, pharmacological compounders are developing products which are 'one shot' ear medications. Thus, for example, BNT otic® contains enrofloxacin, triamcinolone, and ketoconazole in a lanolin anhydrous base, which absorbs water. Similarly, Polox A Gel Otic® contains a similar spectrum of medicants in a preparation which is liquid while refrigerated but firms upon reaching body temperature into a gel which fills the external ear canal. Otic Armor's Liquid bandage® is a residual (up to 3 month's activity claimed) which fills the external ear canal with a water permeable medicated polymer, designed to prevent reinfection.

CHRONIC OR RECURRENT OTITIS EXTERNA IN DOGS

KEY POINTS

- Most cases of chronic otitis externa are bilateral.
- Defects in keratinization, hypersensitivities, and otitis media are the most common causes of chronic, or recurrent, otitis externa.
- Less common causes include allergic contact dermatitis and multiresistant micro-organisms.
- Chronic otitis externa is usually either ceruminous or erythematous and hyperplastic.
- Surgery will be necessary unless chronic pathological change can be prevented or reversed.

History and signalment

From a practical point of view, recurrent otitis externa and chronic otitis externa present similar problems. Indeed, given that relapsing otitis externa will eventually result in chronic disease, the former could be viewed as an early stage of the latter. Both conditions have the potential for inducing irreversible, pathological changes within the external ear canal, and in both instances the clinician is required to institute a diagnostic work-up in order to identify the underlying or predisposing cause(s).

Many breeds are predisposed to chronic otitis externa and clinicians should 'flag' even the first episode as a possible harbinger of future problems. Thus, Cocker Spaniels are not only predisposed from an anatomical point of view but also from the frequency with which defects in keratinization and ceruminous otitis externa occur. Similarly, atopic West Highland White Terriers are predisposed. Larger breeds (Basset Hounds with seborrhoea and Labrador Retrievers with atopy, for example) appear to have some resistance to the onset of chronic pathological changes, perhaps because the external ear canals are much wider and the local microclimate less subject to change. On the other hand, German Shepherd Dogs are notorious for developing chronic obstructive otitis externa, even though they have wide external ear canals and erect pinnae.

Physical examination

Some animals will severely traumatize the area around the pinnae and erythema, alopecia, and crusting may be detected. Similarly, dogs with chronic otitis externa will develop hyperpigmentation and lichenification in the periaural region (Figure 5.5). Affected dogs should be given a thorough examination in an attempt to identify whether the otitis is associated with dermatological lesions. The type of change within the external ear canal may give a pointer to the pattern of dermatological lesion to look for, although clinicians should not be too dogmatic about this as cross-over occurs.

In a dog with ceruminous otitis (Figures 5.6–5.8) the clinician should search for evidence of defects in keratinization and endocrinopathies. Accumulations of greasy scale around the nipples (Figure 5.9), comedones, follicular casts on hair shafts (Figure 5.10), and erythema, perhaps with greasy scale, in the ventral neck folds, axillae, and groin suggest a defect in keratinization. There may be scale, crust (Figure 5.11), and even alopecia on the dorsal trunk. There may be secondary pyoderma and *M. pachydermatis* infection.

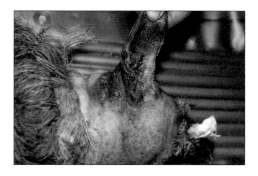

Fig. 5.5 Hyperpigmentation around the base of the pinna and the opening to the external ear canal in this terrier with chronic otitis externa.

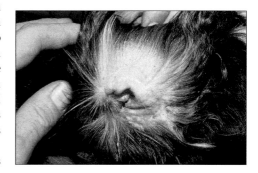

Fig. 5.6 Moderate ceruminous otitis externa in a Cavalier King Charles Spaniel. Note the greasy scale adhering to the surrounding hair.

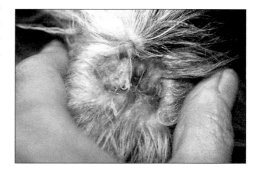

Fig. 5.7 Moderate ceruminous otitis externa in a German Shepherd Dog with a Sertoli cell tumour.

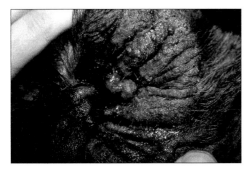

Fig. 5.8 Severe hyperplasia and chronic ceruminous otitis externa.

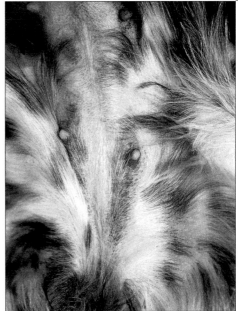

Fig. 5.9 Greasy scale adhering around the nipples. Note also the comedones.

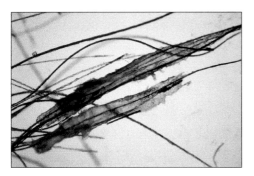

Fig. 5.10 Follicular casts adhering to hair shafts. Follicular casts reflect abnormal follicular keratinization.

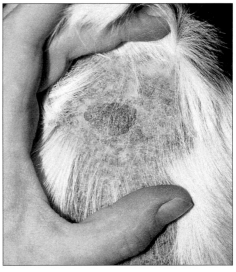

Fig. 5.11 Erythema, alopecia, and patches of crust in a Cocker Spaniel with a defect in keratinization.

In a dog with erythematous hyperplastic changes (Figures 5.12–5.14) characteristic of hypersensitivity, the clinician should look for similar changes on the concave aspect of the pinnae (Figure 5.15), in the dorsal and plantar interdigitae (Figure 5.16), on the flexor aspect of the carpus (Figure 5.17), and on the extensor aspect of the tarsus. In addition, the coat may be rather harsh and dry and be accompanied by a fine scale. There may be a secondary superficial pyoderma and *M. pachydermatis* infection.

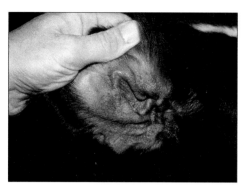

Fig. 5.12 Erythematous, hyperplastic otitis externa in a Rottweiler.

Fig. 5.13 Erythematous, hyperplastic otitis externa.

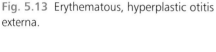

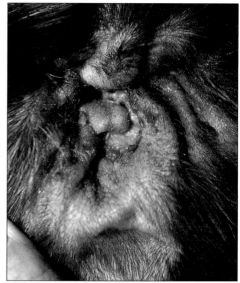

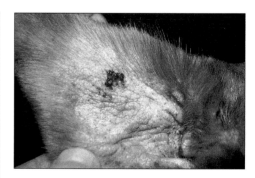

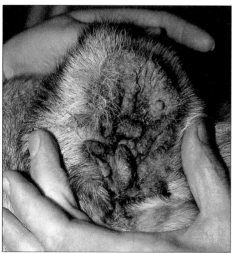

Fig. 5.14 Erythematous, hyperplastic otitis has continued in this German Shepherd Dog with atopy, even though the dog has been subject to lateral wall resection.

Fig. 5.15 Erythematous, hyperplastic changes on the concave aspect of the pinna in a dog with atopy.

Otic examination and other investigations

Most cases of chronic or recurrent otitis externa manifest some degree of hyperplasia of the epithelial lining of the external ear canal (Figure 5.18). Although this may be not be readily apparent on gross examination, it will be visible on histopathological examination of biopsy samples. The epithelial lining may appear grossly normal or may have a cobblestone-like pattern (Figure 5.19)

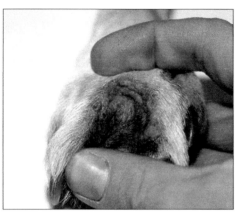

Fig. 5.16 Hyperpigmentation following chronic inflammation in the interdigital areas of a Labrador Retriever with atopy.

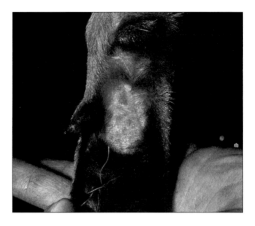

Fig. 5.17 Discrete patch of erythema and alopecia immediately distal to the accessory carpal pad on the plantar aspect of the distal limb of a German Shepherd Dog with atopy.

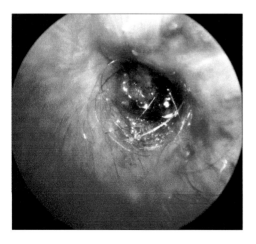

Fig. 5.18 Otoscopic picture of the external ear canal of an atopic dog. Note the erythema and early hyperplasia.

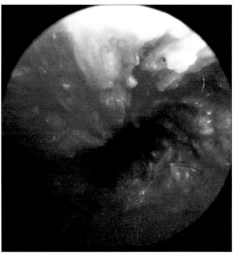

Fig. 5.19 Otoscopic picture of more advanced hyperplastic changes in an external ear canal; the 'cobblestone' pattern is clearly visible.

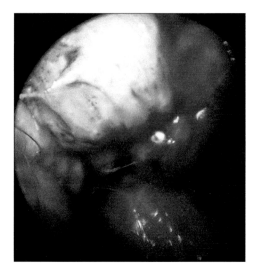

Fig. 5.20 Otoscopic view of an external
ear canal almost completely obstructed by
hyperplastic epithelium.

if glandular and epithelial hyperplasia is
present. In some cases the canal may be
stenosed by proliferative epithelial changes
(Figure 5.20), which are often localized or
polyploid in the cat. Epithelial hyperplasia
and accumulation of cerumen may result
in complete obstruction of the horizontal
canal. The deeper portion of the horizontal
ear canal and tympanum is completely
hidden from view and protected from
topical treatment – 'false middle ear'.

Attempting to classify the changes
within the ear canal as ceruminous or
erythematous hyperplastic, is helpful
from a management point of view. However, the basic elements of the otic examination should still be carried out. Given
that many of these animals will have a

degree of stenosis within the canal and
that all are at risk for concurrent otitis
media, the investigation should probably
be performed under sedation so that
radiography of the bullae, and advanced
diagnostic imaging (where available),
assessment of the tympanum and, possibly,
myringotomy can be performed.

Otoscopic examination may reveal large
quantities of ceruminous discharge in
some cases (Figures 5.21, 5.22); in other ears
there may be minimal discharge. Air-dried
smears should be examined unstained
and after staining with Diff-Quik (Figures
5.23–5.25). Yeast and bacteria may be
identified, in addition to cellular elements
and variably proteinaceous exudate.

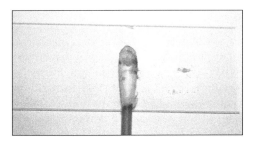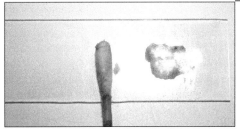

Figs. 5.21, 5.22 Photographs of air-dried cerumen from normal (**5.21**) and ceruminous-type (**5.22**) ear canals demonstrating the breadth of appearance of the sample.

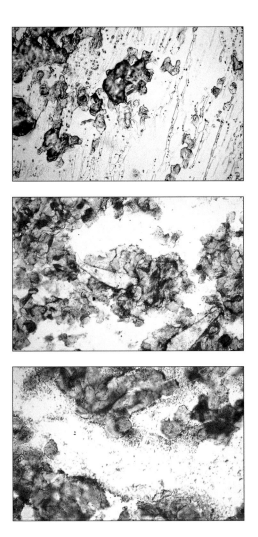

Figs. 5.23–5.25 Photomicrographs of cerumen from a hyperplastic-type ear canal. Ceruminous debris and microbes are clearly apparent and there are no inflammatory cells.

Not all exudate contains pathogenic micro-organisms. Microscopic examination of otic exudate only allows identification of the relative number and physical classification of organisms; yeast, coccus, bacillus, gram positive, or gram negative, for example. The presence of a neutrophilic infiltrate may suggest an infectious process, or at least that inflammation is present. Absence of such an inflammatory infiltrate might strongly suggest that any micro-organisms are nonpathogenic and that any discharge relates to ceruminous gland hyperactivity (which can be prodigious) and epithelial hyperproliferation, rather than to infection. Histopathological examination of biopsy samples may be useful in identifying the degree of fibrosis present (Figures 5.26, 5.27). Topical glucocorticoids may be useful in suppressing mural oedema and hyperplasia, provided fibrosis is minimal.

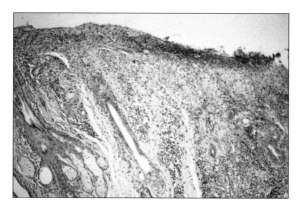

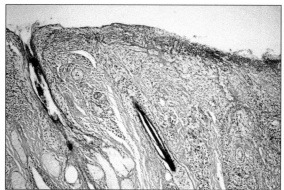

Figs. 5.26, 5.27 Photomicrographs of histopathological samples from a case of chronic otitis externa. Epidermal hyperplasia, an inflammatory infiltrate, and dermal oedema (**5.26**). The same section but stained to highlight fibrosis (**5.27**). This degree of fibrosis is not amenable to topical glucocorticoids; surgery rather than medicine is indicated.

Use of glucocorticoids to treat chronic change

A careful assessment of the ear canal and middle ear should be undertaken in all cases of chronic disease to decide if the ear is irreversibly damaged or whether it can still be managed with medical therapy. Some of the situations where the damage is deemed irreversible include:

- Where the canal is stenotic and the walls are calcified.
- Where severe ceruminous gland hyperplasia is present.
- Where hearing tests (brainstem evoked auditory evoked responses) reveal the dog to be deaf.
- Where there is severe damage to the middle ear identified on radiographs or advanced diagnostic techniques.

Where changes are less severe rational use of glucocorticoids can be undertaken to try to reverse changes within the canal. It is important to have infection controlled before embarking on an extended course of glucocorticoids.

Glucocorticoids can be administered in a range of ways and several methods may be used in combination at the discretion of the clinician:

- Potent topical glucocorticoids (dexamethasone, betamethasone, mometasone, or hydrocortisone aceponate) in a licensed otic drop may be administered when the ear drum is intact, or off-licensed injectable dexamethasone (2 mg/ml) may be mixed with a flush solution e.g. EDTA-tris when the ear drum is ruptured.

- Systemic glucocorticoids may be given orally, e.g. prednisolone at a dose of 1 mg/kg daily for 14 days then on an alternate day basis for a further 2 weeks.
- Glucocorticoids may be administered in ear wicks. The same procedure should be followed as described above in the treatment of infectious otitis externa with ear wicks, but the wick may be soaked with a combination of antibiotic and glucocorticoids or glucocorticoids alone. Dexamethasone 2 mg/ml injectable solution is suitable to soak the wick. The wick may be left *in situ* for 7–10 days before being removed and, if necessary, replaced after flushing of the ear.
- Localized injection of glucocorticoid directly into the wall of the canal may also be used. This is best accomplished using the high magnification lens of the video-otoscope. A flexible hollow needle can be inserted down the working channel of the otoscope or a long spinal needle can be inserted into the canal alongside the otoscope to inject small blebs of glucocorticoid into the canal or into specific lesions. A total volume of 0.5–1.0 ml may be injected into each ear canal depending on the degree of change and the size of the dog.

6 OTITIS MEDIA

AETIOLOGY

Otitis media is common and is almost invariably accompanied by otitis externa[1–3]. Furthermore, in the vast majority of cases the infection within the middle ear appears to result from extension of otitis externa, rather than from ascending infection via the auditory tube or as a result of haematogenous infection[1]. However, it may be that the role of the auditory tube in the aetiology of canine otitis media has not been fully appreciated, since its normal physiological role is critical to middle ear homeostasis, both microbiological and environmental[4,5]. Most cases of otitis media appear to be missed, since in one study the duration of the condition, before diagnosis, was in excess of 2 years in over one-half of cases[3].

The micro-organisms isolated from cases of otitis media are principally those associated with otitis externa, i.e. *Staphylococcus pseudintermedius*, *Pseudomonas* spp., *Proteus* spp., *Escherichia coli*, and *Malassezia pachydermatis*[1,2]. However, aerobic bacteria were isolated from nearly one-half of the normal middle ears sampled in one study[6], suggesting a normal flora, presumably derived from pharyngeal flora ascending the auditory tube. The bacteria recovered were principally *E. coli*, staphylococci, and *Branhamella* spp., together with yeast[6].

Otitis media usually results as an extension of otitis externa through the tympanum, which may subsequently heal, even in the presence of otitis media. How-ever, the bacteria recovered from behind an intact tympanum in cases of otitis media are not always the same species, or with the same antibacterial sensitivity, as those within the external ear canal[2]. Bacteria (especially *S. pseudintermedius* and *Pseudomonas* spp.) and yeast were most commonly found in the external ear canal, whereas bacteria alone were more common in the middle ear. A greater variety of bacteria, including anaerobes, Group D streptococci, and *E. coli*, were found in the middle ear compared to the external ear canal[2].

Other causes, particularly of unilateral otitis media, include foreign bodies which have penetrated the tympanum, inflammatory polyps (especially in cats), and neoplasms such as fibromas and squamous cell carcinomas[1].

The pathological changes within the infected middle ear were reported by Little *et al.*[7]. All the cases in their study were accompanied by pathological changes within the external ear canal, supporting the theory of an association between the two conditions. There was epidermal hyperplasia with a replacement of the normal stratified squamous epithelium by pseudostratified columnar type. The underlying dermis was infiltrated by a mixed inflammatory cell population and it took on the appearance of granulation tissue, occasionally with spicules of bone within it. Secretory cells and gland-like structures appeared within this inflamed granulation tissue. Most of the tympanic membranes were thickened.

Cholesteatomas

Cholesteatomas are slowly enlarging, cystic lesions within the middle ear cavity. They are lined by stratified squamous epithelium and keratin squames are shed into them. They are thought to arise when a pocket of the tympanic membrane contacts, and adheres to, inflamed mucosa within the middle ear[7]. Cholesteatomas are associated with chronic otitis externa, particularly if there is marked stenosis, or even total occlusion, of the external ear canal. In addition to otitis externa they may be associated with local pain, pain when eating, and head tilt[7]. Radiographically, cholesteatomas are associated with increased density within the middle ear cavity and disruption or a change in shape of the middle ear cavity. There is usually stenosis and calcification of the external ear canal[7].

CLINICAL SIGNS

The most common clinical signs associated with otitis media are those of otitis externa or, rarely, of otitis interna[1,8,9]. Pain may be a feature in some cases and animals may resent patting of the aural region or may exhibit frantic head shaking (Figure 6.1). Dogs may have problems chewing hard food or carrying a ball or toy due to pain in the region of the temporo-mandibular joint. Otitis externa is often present and animals commonly have a history of chronic or recurrent otitis externa[8]. Neurological signs are unusual but include head tilt (Figure 6.2), ataxia, Horner's syndrome (Figure 6.3), or facial nerve paralysis (Figures 6.4, 6.5)[7,9,10]. Keratoconjunctivitis sicca may, rarely, result from otitis media, following damage to the parasympathetic innervation of the lachrymal gland[9].

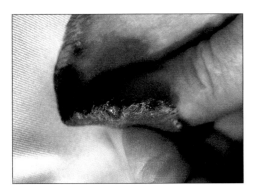

Fig. 6.1 Pinnal trauma as a consequence of otitis media. This dog displayed incessant head shaking.

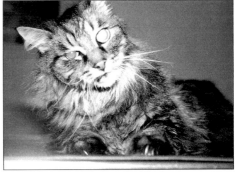

Fig. 6.2 Dramatic head tilt to the right in a domestic longhaired cat with peripheral vestibular disease associated with otitis media.

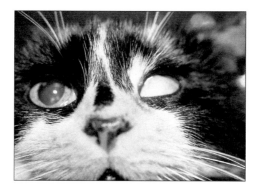

Fig. 6.3 Horner's syndrome on the left-hand side. The markedly prolapsed third eyelid prevents examination of the pupil. This cat had a nasopharyngeal polyp which passed through the middle ear, then through the tympanic membrane into the external ear canal where it produced signs of an obstructive otitis externa.

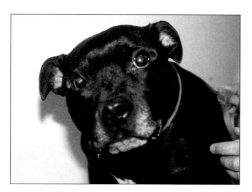 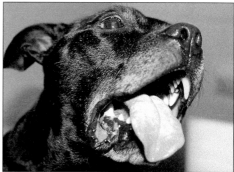

Figs. 6.4, 6.5 Horner's syndrome and facial nerve paralysis in a Staffordshire Bull Terrier. There is right-sided head tilt, a myotic right pupil, and facial paralysis resulting in drooping of the lips on the right-hand side of the face.

Otitis interna may occur following extension of infection into the inner ear via the oval window. Signs of otitis interna include[1,8]: deafness, head tilt and circling toward the affected side, nystagmus with the fast component away from the affected side, and asymmetrical ataxia.

MAJOR DIFFERENTIAL DIAGNOSES

Idiopathic canine and feline vestibular syndromes are the most common nonmiddle ear disorders associated with peripheral vestibular signs[10]. However, in contrast to otitis media these diseases usually show signs of gradual clinical improvement in 1–10 days[10].

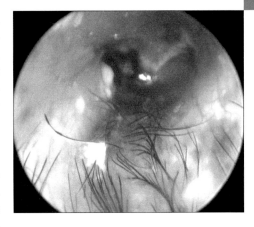

Fig. 6.6 Otoscopic view of a thickened and ruptured tympanic membrane.

DIAGNOSIS

Otoscopy

Otoscopy has good specificity but poor sensitivity[11]. Otitis media should be suspected in all cases of chronic otitis externa or in cases with recurrent episodes of otitis externa. The presence of a ruptured tympanic membrane is diagnostic (Figure 6.6). However, the presence of inflammation and exudate within the external ear canal makes meaningful examination of the tympanum difficult[11]. When the ear drum is ruptured a sample may be taken directly from the middle ear. This can be achieved by inserting a clean otoscope cone or video-otoscope head into the canal as far into the horizontal canal as possible and inserting a fine catheter or a micro-swab through the tube or working channel to 'guard' it from discharge from the external canal. Material can be gathered onto the swab or suctions up the catheter to sample the middle ear. The presence of an intact tympanum does not rule out otitis media since the defect in the tympanum often heals, even in the presence of ongoing otitis media[2]. These complications make definitive otoscopic diagnosis difficult. However, myringotomy can be employed to take samples from the middle ear if the tympanum is intact.

Myringotomy

Surgical incision of the intact tympanum (myringotomy) is indicated in a number of instances:

- To obtain samples of the effusion within the middle ear cavity for microbial culture and sensitivity testing, if otitis media is present.
- To provide a route of access to, or drainage of, accumulated middle ear effusion.
- To provide a means of access to the middle ear cavity to permit flushing, or to facilitate instillation of medication or insertion of a transtympanic ventilation tube.
- Myringotomy must be carried out under direct visual observation.
- The external ear canal must be carefully cleaned and dried before myringotomy is performed.

Needle aspiration

Given that different organisms with different antibacterial sensitivity patterns may exist either side of an intact tympanic membrane[2], it may be necessary to obtain samples from the middle ear by puncturing the intact tympanum and aspirating its contents.

A 22 gauge spinal needle[2] or a paediatric scalp vein catheter are suitable since both are of an appropriate length to be passed through an otoscope. The catheter must be carried to the tympanum by fine-nosed crocodile forceps; this has the advantage of providing a more flexible connection to the 5 ml or 10 ml syringe which is required to aspirate the middle ear contents[2,9].

There are two disadvantage of simple paracentesis[12]. Firstly, the effusion within the middle ear is often purulent or particulate and narrow needles may become blocked; subsequently, trying to pass even a small swab through the first hole is nigh on impossible. Secondly, the puncture is too small and it heals too quickly to permit adequate drainage of any effusion.

Incisional myringotomy

Greater access may be required for drainage or instillation of medication. Two types of incision are recommended: curvilinear or radial[12]. Both are made into the inferior, caudal quadrant of the tympanum using a Gerzog and Sexton or Buck myringotomy knife. Prior to myringotomy, radiographs of the middle ears should be taken to assess the degree of effusion. Tympanometry may also be helpful as abnormal thickening of the tympanum may be detected and this may have implications in that myringotomy may be more difficult and healing may be compromised. Care must be taken not to incise the tympanum too deeply as structures of the middle and inner ear may be damaged. Similarly, too forceful flushing should be avoided. Postmyringotomy antibacterial cover is indicated until the tympanic defect has healed. Surgical defects in the tympanum of experimental dogs showed evidence of healing by 10 days but this was not complete until 21–35 days postsurgery[13].

Curvilinear incision provides better drainage than a radial incision[12]. Using a myringotomy knife, a curved incision is made parallel to, but away from, the periphery of the tympanum (Figure 6.7). Radial incision allows poorer examination of the middle ear than curvilinear incision and makes removal of inspissated material, in particular, difficult[12].

Wire-mounted, small pharyngeal swabs provide an ideal method of collecting samples for microbiology as they are flexible, do not break, and are small enough to permit direct visual manipulation through the otoscope. Once the laboratory sample is collected the effusion may be drained with a blunt needle or washed out with repeated cycles of flushing with a warmed, aqueous solution of an antibacterial agent.

Imaging the middle ear

Radiographic examination of the middle ear cannot always demonstrate changes consistent with otitis media, giving false-negative findings compared to surgery in 25–30% of cases[14,15]. False-positive radiographic findings generally do not occur when compared with surgical diagnosis[14,15]. In an effort to minimize false-negative results, clinicians and imagers have investigated other techniques, in particular computed tomography (CT) and magnetic resonance imaging (MRI).

Radiography

Radiographic techniques have good specificity but poor sensitivity, being able to delineate soft tissue, fluid, or bony changes within the middle ear in only about 70% of cases[10]. They are particularly useful in evaluation of bone involvement (e.g. petrous temporal bone) and in cases where neoplasia is suspected[14]. The open-mouth views are most useful[14], although in a series of cases in which otitis media persisted after bulla osteotomy the lateral oblique view was superior[14,16]. The normal bullae have an identifiable air density within the tympanic cavity. Otitis media results in increased soft tissue density within the bullae (Figures 6.8, 6.9) and, if present, is a reliable indicator of disease within the middle ear[1,14]. Positive contrast ear canalography may also be used to demonstrate otitis media[17].

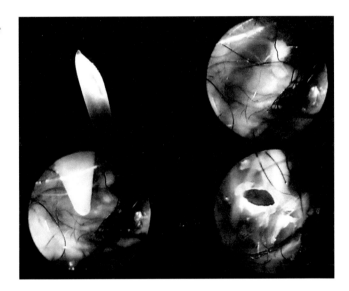

Fig. 6.7 Myringotomy. Note that the controlled incision avoids both the periphery and the manubrium. (Courtesy of Dr. LN Gottelf, with permission of *Waltham Focus*.)

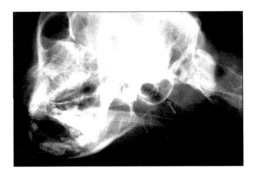
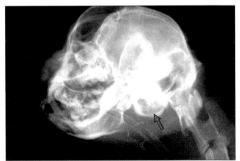

Figs. 6.8, 6.9 Lateral oblique views of the tympanic bullae of a 3-year-old Himalayan cat with left-sided otitis media associated with a nasopharyngeal polyp. Compare Fig. **6.8** (normal bulla, arrow) and Fig. **6.9** (soft tissue density within the bulla, arrow).

Computed tomography

CT has a resolution somewhat less than conventional radiography and it takes much longer to perform, in the order of 20–30 minutes[14,15,18]. However, by taking repeated, sequential views in the same plane, and then using computed processing, it is possible, digitally, to remove extraneous superimposed structures, permitting visualization of the middle and inner ear[18] (Figures 6.10, 6.11).

Precise positioning and an absolute minimum of movement are prerequisites for CT[18]. Animals are placed in ventral recumbency and they must be under general anaesthesia to minimize movement[18]. In one study, which compared CT with radiography in the diagnosis of otitis media[15], CT gave 11% false positives and 17% false negatives (compared to surgical diagnosis), making the technique more sensitive but somewhat less specific than radiography[14]. Neither radiography nor

CT was able to detect early changes of otitis media where there was no osseous change.

The authors of one study, which compared radiography with CT in the diagnosis of otitis media, concluded that CT gave too little additional information to justify the additional logistical and financial costs incurred[15].

Magnetic resonance imaging

MRI uses a completely different principle to radiography and CT[19,20] and the images which result are best regarded as complementary to, rather than replacements for, CT. Thus, CT gives better definition of osseous changes than MRI, whereas the latter gives better definition of soft tissue lesions than CT[21] (Figure 6.12).

MRI has been used in the diagnosis of otitis media in dogs, although only one case report exists to date[22]. One experimental study investigated the potential of MRI to assess otitis media in chinchillas and cats[23].

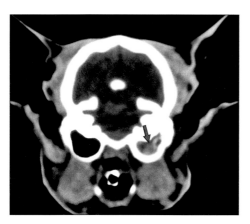

Fig. 6.10 CT scan of a cat with otitis media. There is an effusion within the bulla.

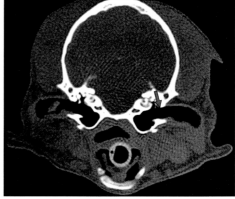

Fig. 6.11 CT scan of a dog with a soft tissue mass within the horizontal ear canal. Note that the mass, a neoplasm, has clearly breached the tympanic membrane (arrow).

The authors reported superior results using T2-weighted images (requiring a 20 minute scanning/measurement cycle) compared to T1-weighted images (taking about 5 minutes). In addition, using a contrast agent (gadolinium-diethylenetriaminepenta-acetic acid) it was possible to visualize inflamed, swollen middle ear mucosa.

In humans, comparative studies in malignant otitis (a particularly severe *Pseudomonas* spp. infection of the external ear canal) and the fine structure of the temporomandibular joint[21,24], found that CT was superior for documenting subtle osseous changes whereas MRI was superior in detecting soft tissue aberrations. Furthermore, in a study comparing CT with MRI in detecting osteoid sarcoma, it was recommended that MR images should not be interpreted without reference to plain radiographs and CT if serious errors in diagnosis were to be avoided[25].

MANAGEMENT

Given that most cases of otitis media are associated with otitis externa, the treatment of the former cannot be considered in isolation from the latter[1,9,10]. The approach to each case should be structured with this in mind.

Flushing and suctioning the bulla

Flushing the bulla is key to successful therapy of otitis media. The mucus and purulent material within the middle ear prevents adequate penetration of topical medication. Hydration of the mucus within the middle ear with a water-based flush makes it less tenacious and easier to suction. The solution to be used to flush the middle ear should be warmed to body temperature before installation. Suitable flush solutions in dogs include water, sterile saline, dilute chlorhexidine solution (<0.2%) and ethylenediamine tetra-acetic

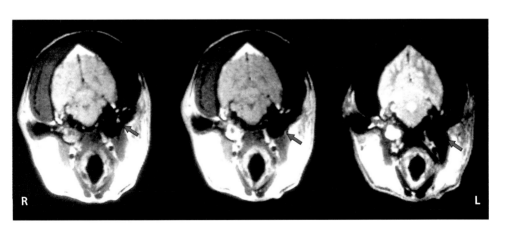

Fig. 6.12 MRI of a cat with left-sided otitis media (arrows). Note that the third image is much clearer: this is the T2-weighted image.

acid tromethamine (EDTA-tris), all of which have been shown to be very safe as flushes even when the ear drum is ruptured[26]. Although ceruminolytics are generally not used as commonly in otitis media due to the nature of the discharge, only squalene has been shown to be safe in the dog[27]. In the cat flushes should be used with care; only water, sterile saline, and EDTA-tris are considered safe. Chlorhexidine has been shown to have ototoxic effects even at low concentrations[28–30].

Tube flushing of the middle ear is the most effective way to clean it. A soft feeding tube or a urinary catheter may be used and can be carefully introduced into the middle ear by sliding it along the floor of the horizontal canal and then directing it ventrally into the tympanic bulla. Where possible the flushing tube should be introduced down the working channel of a video-otoscope to allow better visualization of the flushing process. Care should be taken to avoid introducing the tube into the dorsal or middle aspects of the middle ear, which may result in damage to the delicate structures of the oval and round window that lie within the promontory. Once the tube has been positioned within the bulla, repeated cycles of fluid infusion and aspiration can be performed until the flush solution removed becomes clear.

Infusing topical medication into the bulla

Once the external ear canal and the middle ear have been successfully cleaned medication can be introduced into the middle ear. This can again be infused down a soft feeding tube or urinary catheter. No medication is licensed for the therapy of otitis media; therefore, when topical medication is infused into the bulla a careful assessment should be made of the risks of the topical drugs causing signs of ototoxicity versus the benefits in resolving

infection (see Chapter 7 Ototoxicity and Other Side-effects of Otic Medication). The safest antibiotics for infusion are fluoroquinolones (ciprofloxacin, enrofloxacin, marbofloxacin)[26,31], aqueous penicillin G[26], and aqueous gentamicin[26,32]. Other aminoglycosides, such as tobramycin and semisynthetic penicillin ticarcillin, have been associated with severe hearing loss when used to treat otitis externa[26]. Antifungal drugs that are considered safe are clotrimazole[26,31], miconazole, nystatin, and tolnaftate[31], although one author (SP) has seen temporary deafness caused by both clotrimazole- and miconazole-based products that resolved when topical medication was withdrawn. The aqueous forms of anti-inflammatory drugs dexamethasone[26,31] and fluocinolone[31] also appear to be safe in the middle ear.

Providing the ear is cleaned adequately prior to application of medication, the use of aqueous nonototoxic drugs directly into the bulla hastens recovery from otitis media. The tympanic bulla of the dog and cat is a deep blind ending 'bucket' so that when a drug is infused in, it cannot escape easily and therefore provides long-acting high-concentration effects. Most drugs are thought to remain in the bulla for several days after infusion[33].

Reducing inflammation with glucocorticoids

Glucocorticoids are important to reduce the inflammation and exudation that is found in middle ear disease. Glucocorticoids help to reverse some of the granulation tissue that forms within the bulla. They also help to reduce the amount and viscosity of the mucus produced by the mucoperiosteum and reduce swelling within the auditory tube, which may help to improve drainage from the tympanic bulla into the nasopharynx[33]. Care should be taken to ensure that the patient is a suitable candidate for glucocorticoid therapy, e.g. no history of demodicosis, diabetes, or pregnancy. Glucocorticoids can be administered in a range of ways depending on the clinician's preference. One author (SP) prefers to administer intravenous dexamethasone (2 mg/ml) at a dose of 0.1–0.2 mg/kg at the time of the ear flush and then follow that up with anti-inflammatory doses of prednisolone 1–2 mg/kg daily by mouth for 2 weeks.

Other systemic glucocorticoids that can be used orally include methylprednisolone 0.8–1.8 mg/kg and triamcinolone acetonide 0.1–0.2 mg/kg. Aqueous dexamethasone or a combination of a commercial product containing dimethylsulfoxide (DMSO)/fluocinolone can also be instilled into the bulla via a catheter at the time of flushing. It is important to warn owners of the side-effects of using prednisolone at such high doses, i.e. polyuria, polydipsia, polyphagia, otherwise they may discontinue therapy before the end of the 2-week course. Where unacceptable side-effects are seen with prednisolone, a second injection of dexamethasone may be given as an alternative. Glucocorticoids should be given for a minimum of 2 weeks before reassessment. At that stage prednisolone may be reduced to an alternate day regime or withdrawn, depending on the response to therapy.

Administer systemic antibiotics

The basis of topical therapy in otitis media is that oral antibiotic levels in the tympanic bulla cannot approach topical levels. However, when topical therapy is unsuccessful due to lack of accessibility of the middle ear, e.g. due to stenosis of the canal or due to excessive discharge preventing adequate penetration of topical medication, systemic medication may be useful.

Oral fluoroquinolones are useful where shown to be appropriate based on culture and sensitivity. The most common orally administered drugs include difloxacin at 5.0–10.0 mg/kg once daily; enrofloxacin 5 mg/kg once daily but may be up to 20 mg/kg once daily; marbofloxacin 2.0–5.5 mg/kg once daily; and orbifloxacin 5–12.5 mg/kg once daily.

Aminoglycosides may also be used systemically; like fluoroquinolones their use should be based on culture and sensitivity testing. All animals should have their renal function assessed before starting systemic aminoglycoside treatment. The development of nephrotoxicity should be monitored by the use of daily urine examination and sequential blood samples in all cases. Drugs which may be used are gentamicin at a dose of 6–8 mg/kg daily subcutaneously; amakacin at a dose of 15–20mg/kg daily subcutaneously. Another drug which may be used systemically is ticarcillin–clavulanic acid given intravenously at a dose of 15–25 mg/kg three times daily[33].

TREATMENT OF NASOPHARYNGEAL POLYPS IN CATS

The key to successful therapy is the removal of the polyp. In most cases polyps can be removed by traction/avulsion. The polyp is grasped using alligator forceps or a grasping tool down the video-otoscope. The polyp is pulled and twisted to tear its attachment away creating minimal haemorrhage. As an alternative to traction, polyps can be removed by carbon dioxide laser ablation.

When cats are treated postoperatively with systemic prednisolone (1–2 mg/kg daily for 2 weeks, then half the initial dose for 1 week, then every other day for a further week before discontinuing) the risk of recurrence is reduced significantly[34].

Where removal is impossible or polyps recur, then a ventral bulla osteotomy should be performed.

PROGNOSIS

If the inflammatory process is identified early, the cause identified, and effective treatment instituted, the prognosis for recovery is good. Minor residual vestibular deficits, such as head tilt or mild ataxia, may persist but the animal soon adapts to the 'new' head position. Neurological signs associated with otitis media, such as facial nerve paralysis and Horner's syndrome, may persist.

Some cases of otitis media (and, indeed, some cases of otitis interna) develop osteomyelitis of the osseous bulla and petrous temporal bone. Occasionally the infection ascends the vestibulocochlear and facial nerves to the brainstem, resulting in a brainstem abscess or meningitis associated with central vestibular signs[2].

INTRODUCTION

KEY POINTS

- Clinical cases of true ototoxicity following medical management of otitis externa are very rare.
- Almost all the risks associated with otopharmacy can be obviated provided the clinician can document an intact tympanic membrane before applying the otopharmaceutical agent.
- Side-effects from otic administration of chemicals include local inflammation, otitis media, vestibular or cochlear damage, and systemic absorption.
- Almost any chemical will cause inflammation within the middle ear or inner ear if instilled through the tympanum.
- The round window is an important portal for the passage of drugs, toxins, and inflammatory mediators from the middle to the inner ear.
- The nonpharmaceutical component of an otic preparation (penetrance enhancer, detergent) may significantly affect the toxic potential of the product.

Many types of medication are applied to the external ear canal of dogs and cats. In addition to specific medications, such as anti-inflammatory agents, acaricides, antimicrobial agents, and ceruminolytics, there may be substances included to enhance penetration and to act as vehicle components and preservatives.

The anatomy of the external ear canal is such that liquid medications, in excess, will tend to pool in the horizontal canal. High concentrations of medication may thus come into contact with inflamed epithelium and the potential for intra- and percutaneous absorption is readily apparent. In some circumstances this is desirable. For example, the anti-inflammatory effect of a topical glucocorticoid must be exerted on dermal tissues. In contrast, an antimicrobial, antifungal, or acaricidal agent will usually be applied to the external ear canal for their topical effect and absorption is not necessary.

Inflammation within, and overt damage to, the tympanic and round window membranes may permit inflammatory mediators or drugs to enter the middle ear or inner ear, respectively. Furthermore, it is not known to what extent penetration enhancers, such as propylene glycol (a common ingredient in otic preparations), may increase the passage of these substances across these membranes.

The unwanted effects of otic medication may be classified into four groups:

- Direct effects on the meatal and tympanic epithelium and underlying dermis.
- Effects within the middle ear.
- Effects on vestibular and cochlear functions (ototoxicity).
- Systemic sequelae of the otic administration of medications.

One of the greatest difficulties facing clinicians is assessing the relevance of experimental studies, particularly if they are performed in another species. Much experimental research into ototoxicity is performed on guinea pigs and chinchillas. It could be argued that these tests are so artificial, and interspecies anatomical and physiological variation is so great, that the conclusions drawn from experimental animals cannot be applied to dogs with clinical ear disease[1]. Merchant et al.[2] demonstrated that chlorhexidine exhibited very little ototoxic effect in dogs, in contrast to experimental studies which reported both vestibular and cochlear toxicity to chlorhexidine in guinea pigs[3,4]. However, in a recent experimental study using guinea pigs and dogs there was a good correlation between the two species[5], suggesting that extrapolation might be valid in some instances.

MEATAL AND TYMPANIC INFLAMMATION

The effects of various constituents of commercial otic pharmaceutical products on the meatal epithelium and the tympanic membrane were studied in an experimental model[6]. Benzalkonium chloride (a quaternary ammonium preservative) produced profound effects such as acanthosis and surface ulceration. A mixed inflammatory infiltrate in the dermis was also noted. Propylene glycol (a solvent and penetrance enhancer) induced acanthosis

and hyperkeratosis but no histopathological evidence of inflammation was noted. Not surprisingly, both products also induced a statistically significant increase in the epidermal mitotic index. Similar effects were exerted on the tympanic epithelium. The only noted effect of topical hydrocortisone was a significant reduction in the epidermal mitotic index. The authors made the point that it was the supposedly 'inactive' components, rather than the pharmacologically active ingredients, of commercial otopharmaceutical products which induced most change. It may be that these iatrogenic inflammatory effects are, in reality, very mild in nature and are probably masked by the more marked changes consequent upon otitis externa. Thus, they may be of little clinical significance. However, until definitive studies are performed this cannot be relied upon.

Otic maceration may result from over-enthusiastic or prolonged application of aqueous or propylene glycol-based cleansers. This might particularly be the case when otic preparations are used for the long-term management of ear disease, such as in allergic otitis externa[7]. Suspicion should be raised when examination of the external ear canal reveals moderate inflammation accompanied by an accumulation of white, moist debris composed of sloughed squames, with no inflammatory cells present.

EFFECTS WITHIN THE MIDDLE EAR

Several types of otic medication can induce inflammation within the middle ear, if they reach it via a ruptured tympanum. Several commercial ceruminolytic preparations were recently shown to cause acute inflammation within the middle ear[5]. Propylene glycol is well documented as an irritant of middle ear epithelium[8].

Chronic inflammation within the middle ear is thought to be associated with cholesteatoma formation[9,10]. Propylene glycol is the main agent used for experimental induction of cholesteatomas[10] and it is a common ingredient in many commercial otic pharmaceuticals. Whether this, or other, chemotherapeutic agents are involved in the induction of cholesteatomas in dogs is not known. However, many polypharmaceutical otic preparations contain glucocorticoids in addition to putative irritants, and intratympanic administration of prednisolone with propylene glycol has been shown to inhibit propylene glycol-induced inflammation and subsequent cholesteatoma formation[10].

OTOTOXICITY

An ototoxic agent produces cochlear or vestibular damage by injuring structures within the inner ear[1,11]. The effects may reflect uni- or bilateral toxicity. Clinical signs of vestibular damage may be reflected very early after the insult has been effected and these include nystagmus, strabismus, ataxia, head tilt, and circling. Clinical signs of cochlear damage usually go unnoticed until complete deafness is recognized[1]. The early signs of cochlear damage in man include tinnitus and although this would be difficult to document in dogs and cats, it may be that an inappropriate, or unusually strong, response to an auditory stimulus is a reflection of early cochlear damage[12].

In order for a drug to exert ototoxicity it must reach the inner ear. This may be the result of haematogenous spread following oral or parenteral dosage. However, more commonly it follows topical application of ototoxic agents into the external ear canal and their subsequent passage into the middle ear via a ruptured tympanum. Subsequent diffusion into the middle ear is enhanced by the presence of otitis media, which induces increased permeability through the round window membrane[13–15]. The round window membrane is an important portal for the passage of inflammatory mediators, toxins, and drugs from the middle ear to the inner ear[15].

The potential for a drug to cause ototoxicity will vary: the vehicle, chemical composition, and concentration of the agent in question; the route, frequency, and duration of administration; the concentrations of other components in the otic preparation used; and, in some cases, concurrent administration of other drugs[12]. In summary:

- Direct instillation of most substances into the inner ear is likely to induce ototoxicity.
- Topical administration into the external ear canal in the presence of a ruptured tympanum and/or otitis media increases the risk of ototoxicity.
- Certain detergents may increase the ototoxic potential of chlorhexidine.
- Certain agents, such as some aminoglycosides, are selectively ototoxic, by whatever route they are administered.
- Loop diuretics potentiate aminoglycoside toxicity by increasing their relative concentration in the endolymph.
- Salicylates may potentiate the toxicity of gentamicin.
- Familial sensitivity to aminoglycoside toxicity has been demonstrated in man[16] and may be relevant in veterinary medicine.

Topical products
Vehicles: propylene glycol

Propylene glycol is a solvent and penetrance enhancer found in many proprietary otic preparations[6]. When instilled into the middle and inner ear in experimental studies it is ototoxic[8,9]. In one study[5] some commercial ceruminolytic preparations were shown to induce inflammatory reaction within the middle ear. Some of the dogs exhibited signs of vestibular damage and altered brainstem auditory evoked response (BAER). Two of the three products which were associated with these changes contained propylene glycol, although whether this was the sole agent responsible for the effects is not clear.

Ear cleaners
Ceruminolytics
Mansfield et al.[5] looked at four commercial ceruminolytic preparations commonly used as ear cleaners to assess their potential ototoxicity. He instilled squalene, dioctyl sodium succinate, carbamide peroxide, and triethanolamine into the middle ear of both guinea pigs and dogs. Only the ear cleaner containing squalene showed no morphological or neurological changes.

Antimicrobial flushing agents
Chlorhexidine
Chlorhexidine is readily available in clinical practice and is frequently used for irrigation of the external ear canal. Care must be taken to ensure that adequate dilution is achieved. If it is formulated too weakly, it loses its antimicrobial potency, particularly against gram-negative bacteria; if formulated too strongly, it is ototoxic[17]. A study by Merchant et al.[2] investigated the ototoxic potential of 0.2% chlorhexidine acetate instilled into canine ears before and after experimental myringotomy. No significant effects were noted, suggesting that at 0.2% concentration, or less, chlorhexidine is safe as an irrigating solution in dogs, even in the presence of a ruptured tympanum. Chlorhexidine does not appear to be safe as a flush in cat's ears: solutions as dilute as 0.05% cause cochlear and vestibular ototoxicity and mucosal injury[18-20].

Aqueous solutions of chlorhexidine (0.15%) combined with ethylenediamine tetra-acetic acid tromethamine (EDTA-tris) also appear to be very safe when used as a middle ear flush[20]. The ototoxicity of chlorhexidine is markedly enhanced in the presence of some, but not all, nonionic or cationic detergents[21,22]. Quaternary ammonium compounds (cetrimide for example) appear to potentiate the toxic effects of chlorhexidine[18] and commercial mixtures of the two compounds (Savlon® for example) should not be instilled into the external ear canal.

Povidone–iodine preparations
Aqueous solutions of certain iodine preparations were found to be nonototoxic in guinea pigs[23] whereas alcohol-based preparations of iodine[23] and povidone–iodine solutions were ototoxic. Both vestibular and cochlear damage was caused.

Acetic acid
A 5% solution of acetic acid (undiluted vinegar) is irritating within the middle ear and should only be used with caution when the tympanum is ruptured[24,25]. Anecdotal reports suggest that a 2–2.5% solution may be safe in the face of a ruptured tympanic membrane[25,26].

EDTA-tris
EDTA-tris is widely available as both a component of commercial ear flushes and as crystals and a ready-to-use aqueous flush. EDTA-tris based products can be used as flushes and presoaks to help potentiate antibiotic therapy or as a carrier vehicle for aminoglycoside and fluoroquinolone antibiotics. EDTA-tris has been widely promoted by many different authorities as a safe and efficacious therapy for otitis media and has rapidly become the treatment of choice for gram-negative otitis externa/media[27-29].

Topical antibacterial agents
Aminoglycosides
Aminoglycosides are common components of topical otic preparations. This group contains amongst others amikacin, framycetin, gentamicin, neomycin, and tobramycin. Many of the studies assessing the topical ototoxicity of this group of drugs have been

performed in guinea pigs and chinchillas. Studies on guinea pigs have shown that neomycin, streptomycin, gentamicin, amikacin, and netilmicin show signs of cochlear toxicity when applied topically into the middle ear[30,31]. One study by Morais demonstrated that the organ of Corti was completely destroyed in guinea pigs after 3 months application of topical neomycin. Similar work in chinchillas has also demonstrated potent topical ototoxicity[32]. Such studies have led to the extrapolation of similar effects in dogs. However, despite fears over the ototoxic potential of gentamicin in dogs, a canine study designed to stimulate clinical exposure via a ruptured tympanic membrane failed to document any noticeable degree of cochlear or vestibular toxicity after 21 days of therapy[33].

Other research looking at BAER testing and neurological assessment of dogs before and after topical administration of drugs into the tympanic bulla[21], demonstrated no signs of ototoxicity when aqueous gentamicin solution was used over a period of 6 weeks. It is therefore possible where reactions to topical gentamicin preparations have been recorded it may have been the vehicle that produced side-effects rather than the antibiotic. Little information is available on the topical ototoxic potential of other aminoglycosides in dogs. The same study which showed that gentamicin was safe in the middle ear demonstrated that an aqueous solution of tobramycin was profoundly ototoxic[21]. To date therefore, the only aminoglycoside that can be used with confidence in the middle ear of the dog is gentamicin.

Fluoroquinolones

Aqueous solutions of fluoroquinolones are widely used in otitis media to treat gram-negative infection. Few studies exist demonstrating their safety, but their widespread use and recommendation by otologists and board certified derma-

tologists has led to them being generally accepted as nonototoxic[24-26,34,35].

Topical application of a 0.2% solution of ciprofloxacin into the middle ear of guinea pigs was shown not to be ototoxic[36]. A BAER study in dogs showed that aqueous solutions of marbofloxacin failed to produce any signs of vestibular or cochlea toxicity[21].

SYSTEMIC EFFECTS OF OTIC MEDICATION

Topically applied drugs pass easily into and through the epithelial lining of the external ear canal. This may be enhanced in the presence of propylene glycol and other agents. The facility of systemic absorption following topical otic administration, even into normal ear canals, is demonstrated by the ability of locally applied glucocorticoid to suppress the pituitary adrenocortical axis[37].

Systemic absorption following topical otic administration may not be limited to glucocorticoids. Measurable serum concentrations of gentamicin occurred in humans and dogs following otic administration[38,39]. Whether the route of absorption was via the epithelium of the external or middle ear, or even if it was via the auditory tube, is not known, although the latter route is unlikely in view of the poor absorption of aminoglycosides via the gut. Given that most topical otic preparations are administered when the otic epithelium is inflamed, it is most probable that absorption was via this route.

OTOTOXICITY OF SYSTEMIC DRUGS

Furosemide, salicylates, and cisplatin and aminoglycoside antibiotics (gentamicin, amikacin) have all been reported to cause ototoxicity in man and experimental animals[1,12]. Aminoglycoside ototoxcity has been recorded in cats after systemic administration of paromomycin for infectious enteritis[40]. Combination of diuretics with aminoglycoside antibiotics or cisplatin in experimental animals and in humans leads to profound permanent hearing loss[41].

SUMMARY

In general, ototoxic effects are dose related, *vis á vis* the middle and inner ear. The first principle, therefore, is to avoid using ototoxic chemicals and, if they must be used, reduce the dose and frequency of administration to an absolute minimum. Careful observation and regular follow-up examinations of the patient may allow detection of vestibular signs early enough to allow the clinician to suspend therapy. In some circumstances prompt action may prevent permanent damage[12]. Unfortunately, it is difficult to detect early cochlear damage[1]. Indeed, it may be virtually impossible to detect unilateral cochlear damage in the clinical setting without recourse to sophisticated investigatory tools, such as BAER.

The use of systemic aminoglycosides such as gentamicin, which are concentrated in the endolymph, should be avoided in the presence of otitis media since inflammation of the round window allows increased penetration of drugs into the inner ear. Concomitant use of loop diuretics should be avoided[11].

With regard to the flushing of the external ear canal, it is best to assume that the tympanum is not intact and to use water, sterile saline, 0.2% chlorhexidine solution, or aqueous EDTA-tris as flushing agents. It is important to remember that certain detergents may potentiate chlorhexidine toxicity and concomitant use should be avoided.

If the tympanum is proven to be intact, cerumenolytics, foamers, and chemical depilatories may be used provided that the ear canal is thoroughly washed, flushed, and dried at the end of the cleaning procedure. Squalene is the only cerumenolytic product that should be used if the ear drum is ruptured.

8 AURAL ABLATION AND BULLA OSTEOTOMY

INTRODUCTION

> ### KEY POINTS
>
> - Surgical ablation of the ear canal is useful in the management of chronic ear disease, provided a critical assessment of the individual case is made on each occasion.
> - Do not underestimate the medical aspects of chronic ear disease. In particular, recognize the contribution that dermatological conditions can make to poor surgical outcome.
> - Total ablation and bulla osteotomy is best performed by an experienced surgeon.
> - Owners should be cautioned that all aural resections, but particularly those involving ablation of the entire vertical canal, may adversely affect ear carriage in dogs with erect pinnae.

The various surgical resections of the external ear canal are generally indicated as a means of resolving chronic otitis externa or as aids in the management of otitis media. The decision on how much of the external ear canal to resect is crucial, since the outcome of the surgical procedure will be assessed by the alleviation of the chronic otitis. For example, failure fully to assess the patient and make a definitive diagnosis of the cause of the otitis externa is the main reason why lateral wall resection fails. Thus, if the underlying cause is atopy or dietary intolerance, the otitis will continue to affect the remaining medial wall of the external ear canal, even after a technically perfect lateral wall resection or vertical canal ablation (Figures 8.1, 8.2).

Surgical management of ear disease cannot be divorced from the medical necessity of fully investigating all the components of the otic structure and recognizing that the epithelial lining of the external ear canal is an extension of the skin of the head and neck. Chronic otitis externa, at least in the dog, is usually a manifestation of a more generalized dermatological process such as a defect in keratinization, hypersensitivity, endocrinopathy, or an immune-mediated disease. Furthermore, many cases are associated with otitis media. These diseases and associated problems must all be fully investigated before surgery is contemplated. Clinicians are urged to read the relevant chapters and sections of this book for further information.

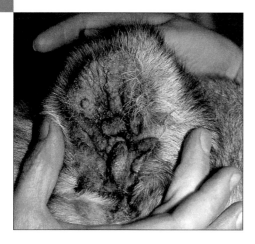

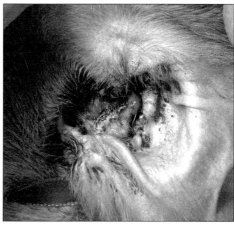

Fig. 8.1 Results of a lateral wall resection in an atopic German Shepherd Dog. The surgeon failed to appreciate that the atopic lesion would continue on the residual lateral and medial walls of the vertical ear canal.

Fig. 8.2 Results of a vertical canal ablation in a German Shepherd Dog. As in the previous case the underlying condition of atopy was not appreciated.

PRESURGICAL INVESTIGATIONS

Presurgical assessment of the entire structure of the ear is essential[1–3]. In many cases some of the procedures advocated below will have been performed by way of routine management and work up of a case of otitis media or externa. A fuller description of these procedures can be found elsewhere in this book.

Palpation of the external ear canal may reveal thickening and ossification of the cartilaginous components. Local thickening, particularly in the parotid area, or the presence of a sinus adjacent to the external ear canal may reflect para-aural abscess[4,5]. Changes to the vertical part of the external ear canal are often accompanied by chronic changes to the concave aspect of the pinna, which may be thickened and lichenified.

Otoscopy is essential and a clear view is mandatory if meaningful conclusions

are to be drawn. Visual examination via an otoscope can provide information on the state of the epithelial lining of the otic canal, the degree of stenosis of the lumen and, sometimes, an indication that neoplasia is present. The status of the tympanic membrane cannot always be assessed fully by otoscopy, even in a normal external ear canal[4].

Neurological examination of the facial, oculosympathetic, and vestibular nerves provides a baseline for assessing the significance of any postoperative neurological signs. Similarly, assessing a dog's auditory ability preoperatively may give a useful measure against which to compare postoperative deafness.

Bacteriological culture and sensitivity testing will often have been performed before surgery is considered. However, repeated use of various topical antibacterial agents may well influence the bacterial population and its antibacterial susceptibility[5]. Preoperative sampling to provide an up-to-date antibacterial susceptibility is advisable if postoperative infection is to be managed effectively[6]. However, if otitis media is present, intra-operative sampling is essential since it has been shown that in the presence of otitis media there is little correlation between the flora of the horizontal ear canal and that of the middle ear[7].

Radiographic assessment of the external ear may reveal ossification of the auricular cartilage and absence of the luminal air shadow, both findings suggestive of chronic, inflammatory, proliferative otitis externa[8,9]. Positive contrast ear canalography may be useful in establishing the status of the tympanum if tympanometry is not available or is impracticable, for instance if the external ear canal is stenosed[8,10]. Radiographic examination of the middle ear is essential in the work up of otitis media[9–11], although ultrasound and computed tomography (CT), perhaps in combination, may be more sensitive for evaluation of otitis media than radiography[12].

Biopsy of the epithelial lining of the external ear canal is rarely performed but, conceivably, it may help to influence whether surgery takes place. For example, if the histopathological pattern is inflammatory, with little evidence of fibrosis and glandular hyperplasia, aggressive glucocorticoid therapy may reduce luminal stenosis, thus obviating the need for surgery. Biopsy of neoplastic lesions may provide information which influences the type of surgical resection required, and it is therefore a useful pre-surgical investigation, particularly if the lesion is accessible. Cytological examination of otic cerumen may help provide information on the tumour type but it cannot grade malignancy; this requires histopathological examination of biopsy samples.

VERTICAL CANAL ABLATION

The purpose of vertical canal ablation is to remove the portion of the external ear canal which contains the most potential for chronic hyperplastic change. In reality, most surgery is performed in patients with irreversible changes already in place, i.e. it is salvage surgery rather than preemptive surgery. Furthermore, most cases of chronic otitis externa exhibit varying degrees of luminal stenosis within the horizontal portion of the external ear canal, in addition to changes within the vertical portion, and in theory this should also be removed. However, the horizontal canal is short and ablation of the vertical canal (provided a good drainplate is fashioned) establishes good drainage, resulting in an improvement of the microenvironment within the remaining portions of the canal. Vertical canal ablation is indicated in the following circumstances[13–15]:

- Chronic, or recurrent, otitis externa associated with irreversible, hyperplastic changes in the luminal epithelium.
- Neoplasia of the vertical ear canal.

Total ear canal ablation (and lateral bulla osteotomy)

Total ear canal ablation (TECA) is always performed with a lateral bulla osteotomy (LBO). The removal of the entire external ear canal can only be accomplished if the external canal is resected to the level of the tympanum, which marks the boundary between the external and the middle ear. This necessitates resection of bone.

TECA and LBO are rarely indicated in cats[2,16]. Although bulla osteotomy alone (usually ventral) may be indicated for the management of polyps, for example, the otitis externa usually resolves and chronic changes are rarely severe enough to warrant vertical canal ablation. TECA and LBO are indicated in the following circumstances[2,3,14,17]:

- Chronic, or recurrent, otitis externa associated with irreversible, hyperplastic changes in the luminal epithelium.
- Failure of more conservative surgery to alleviate otitis externa or media.
- Neoplasia of the external ear canal.
- Otitis media.

Vertical ear canal ablation

The crucial steps in this procedure are:
- Construction of an effective drainplate.
- Careful closure of all dead space.

An initial 'T'-shaped incision is made. The lower point of the incision, the base of the 'T', is just below the level of the horizontal portion of the external ear canal[3,17–19]. The bar of the 'T' follows a circumferential path across the medial wall of the conchal cartilage (Figure 8.3), immediately dorsal to the large antihelicine tubercle[13]. In dogs with erect pinnae, a dorsally curved

incision may be performed; this results in a crescent-shaped base for the pinna and helps to maintain a normal carriage postoperatively[20].

Incision through the auricular cartilage is made, taking care not to penetrate the lateral aspect of the pinna. The 'trumpet' of conchal cartilage is grasped with tissue forceps and a combination of blunt and sharp dissection is used to isolate the vertical canal, which can be pulled free from the underlying tissues (Figure 8.4). It is essential to keep the dissection as close to the cartilage as possible as this minimizes iatrogenic damage to blood vessels and nerves.

The excised canal is sectioned above the level of the horizontal canal to allow creation of a drainplate (Figure 8.5). The ligamentous connection between the annular and conchal cartilages is used as a hinge to allow reflection of the cartilage, as in the lateral wall resection described above. At the new acoustic meatus, exact closure of skin to canal epithelium

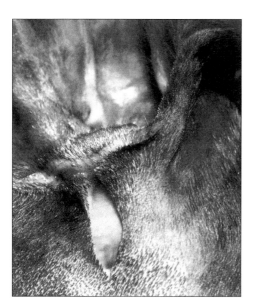

Fig. 8.3 Vertical canal ablation. A 'T'-shaped incision is made over the vertical ear canal.

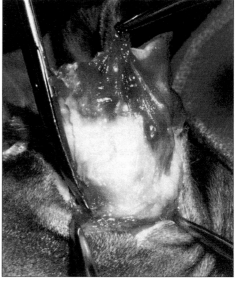

Fig. 8.4 Circumferential dissection of the soft tissues is performed keeping as close to the cartilaginous ear canal as possible.

with 4/0 absorbable monofilament subcuticular sutures is attempted so as to minimize stricture at the site (Figure 8.6). Skin sutures are placed if necessary. The suture line is closed above the drainplate (Figure 8.7), incorporating subcutaneous tissues deep to the excised conchal cartilages with the sutures to eliminate dead space[13]. Failure to close dead space may result in postoperative dehiscence.

Fig. 8.5 The base of the freed vertical ear canal is resected at a level below the diseased tissue, at the level of the horizontal ear canal.

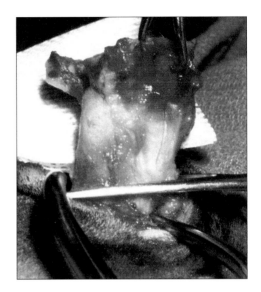

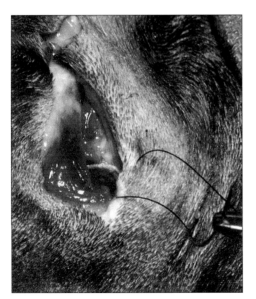

Fig. 8.6 A permanent stoma is constructed by ensuring that the cartilaginous portion of the horizontal ear canal remains patent when sutured to the skin.

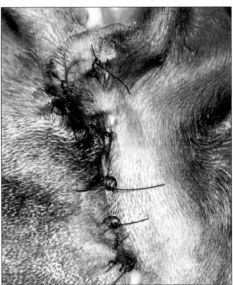

Fig. 8.7 The rest of the incision is closed, ensuring that dead space is eliminated.

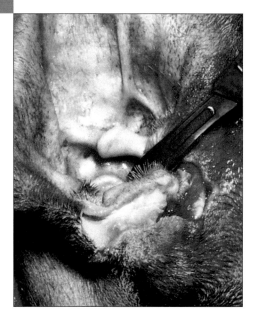

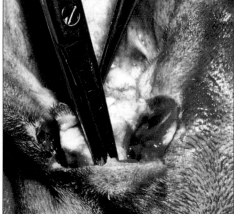

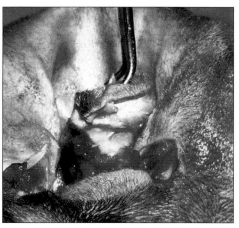

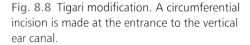
Fig. 8.8 Tigari modification. A circumferential incision is made at the entrance to the vertical ear canal.

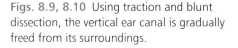
Figs. 8.9, 8.10 Using traction and blunt dissection, the vertical ear canal is gradually freed from its surroundings.

Pull-through modification[21]

This modification of vertical canal ablation results in less incised tissue to suture than with standard techniques, less trauma to subcutaneous tissues, less risk of damage to associated structures such as the salivary glands, less postoperative discomfort, fewer sutures, more rapid healing, and less dead space. Although the original authors did not describe the creation of a drainplate, it is generally considered appropriate to do so.

The circumferential incision is identical to that described above except that a subsequent vertical incision is not made (Figure 8.8). Instead, the conchal cartilage is gradually worked free by digital and blunt dissection until the entire 'trumpet' of the

vertical canal is freed from its soft tissue attachments and exposed via the dorsal incision (Figures 8.9, 8.10).

The skin is palpated at the level of the horizontal canal (Figure 8.11) and a circular incision, roughly one and a half times the diameter of the horizontal canal, is made (Figure 8.12).

The entire, exposed conchal cartilage 'trumpet', which was previously exposed by blunt dissection, is pulled through this ventral incision (Figure 8.13) and cut 1.5 cm (0.6 in) above the level of the horizontal canal (Figure 8.14).

A drainplate is constructed as described above (Figure 8.15) and the distal incision closed (Figure 8.16).

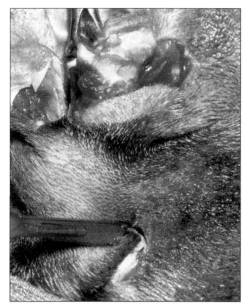

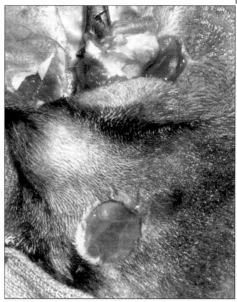

Fig. 8.11 The level of the horizontal ear canal is palpated.

Fig. 8.12 The skin is incised at the level of the horizontal ear canal.

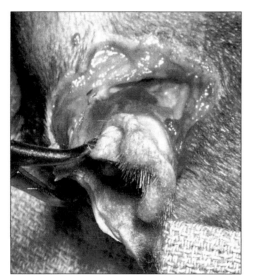

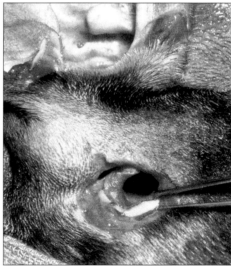

Fig. 8.13 The entire, already freed, conchal cone is pulled through the incision.

Fig. 8.14 The exposed vertical ear canal is excised at the level of the horizontal ear canal.

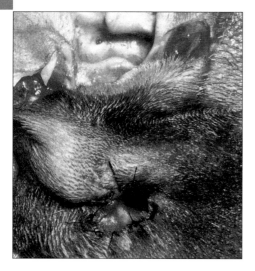

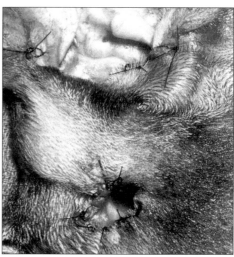

Fig. 8.15 The stoma at the horizontal ear canal is closed, taking care to ensure that the drainplate keeps the opening patent.

Fig. 8.16 The initial circumferential incision is closed in a routine manner.

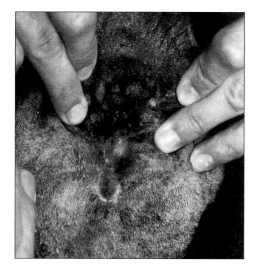

Fig. 8.17 Stenosis of the horizontal ear canal following inadequate construction of the drainplate. The problem was exacerbated by a failure to identify underlying atopy, which resulted in ongoing disease in the remnants of the vertical ear canal and concave aspect of the pinna.

Postoperative care

Postoperative analgesia is mandatory. Postoperative antibacterial therapy should be continued for at least 10 days, or until the sutures are removed[14].

Postsurgical problems

Postsurgical complications with this technique are much less common than those seen after lateral wall resection[13,14,19]. Furthermore, improper patient selection occurs less frequently than with lateral wall resection[17]. In one study[19], dehiscence of the suture line occurred in 12% of cases, with stenosis of the external acoustic meatus occurring in 7% of cases. Damage to the facial nerve is possible, particularly if deep sectioning of the external acoustic meatus is attempted. Stenosis of the external acoustic meatus (Figure 8.17) is usually a consequence of inadequate construction of the drainplate, resulting in a failure to support the canal and impairment of natural drainage[19].

Postsurgical problems can be addressed as follows:

- Postoperative, acute, inflammatory stenosis of the external acoustic meatus may be suppressed if the lumen is packed with glucocorticoid-impregnated gauze for a few days[13].
- Dehiscence is best treated aggressively with systemic antibacterial agents and drainage[19,22]. Consideration should be given to obtaining a culture and sensitivity report if dehiscence occurs in dogs receiving postoperative antibacterial therapy. Surgical closure is indicated as soon as infection is under control[6].
- Stenosis of, or impaired drainage from, the external acoustic meatus warrants investigation since it implies one of two problems, neither mutually antagonistic: inadequate drainplate construction or ongoing otitis media.

Ossification of the external ear canal

Mineralization of the cartilaginous components of the external ear canal may occur as a consequence of chronic inflammation[23]. The initial changes appear to occur in the horizontal canal[23], although with time, and in particular in Cocker Spaniels, the vertical canal may also become ossified. Although the ossified vertical canal may be removed relatively easily by ablation, the surgical resection of ossified horizontal canals is more difficult.

A surgical technique has been described for dissecting out the ossified portions of the horizontal and vertical canals[23,24], although if the condition has progressed to this stage, total ablation and bulla osteotomy may be indicated. However, since total ablation and bulla osteotomy sometimes results in loss of hearing, owners may want to avoid such a radical step, particularly if the contralateral ear has already been ablated.

Although the pain associated with chronic otitis externa was largely controlled in the dogs subjected to this procedure[24], most required occasional treatment to clean the ear canals.

The technique for dissecting out the ossifications is as follows (after Hobson[23] and Elkins et al.[24]):

- If the vertical canal is still present (and is to be ablated, as described above), it is exposed and the dissection is continued ventrally to expose the ventral wall of the ossified horizontal canal, taking great care to avoid the facial nerve.
- In the presence of an ossified vertical canal, ronguers are used to remove ossified cartilage from the lateral surface of that portion of the vertical canal destined to form the drainplate. In effect, the drainplate is constructed from the epithelial components of the vertical canal rather than from the cartilaginous portion.
- An incision is made on the distal aspect of the junction of the annular and auricular cartilages. This allows an osteotome (or a small rounded periosteal elevator) gradually to elevate the soft tissue lining of the horizontal canal. The ossified cartilage can then be gradually removed with ronguers while leaving the soft tissue lining of the ear canal intact.
- Once the ossified material has been removed a drainplate is created from the remnants of the lateral wall of the vertical canal, taking care to ensure that the horizontal canal is patent.

Total ear canal ablation and lateral bulla osteotomy

The crucial steps in this procedure are:

- Avoid damage to the round window and the facial nerve.
- Ensure that all secretory epithelium is removed from the bulla and from the site of the horizontal ear canal.
- Treat tissues gently; ensure good haemostasis and close all dead space.

It is now generally accepted that it is prudent to perform a LBO with every TECA[15,25-27]. Given the difficulty of definitively documenting otitis media by radiography[8], or even by CT[28] (see Chapter 2 for discussion on imaging the bulla), it is almost impossible to justify not performing a bulla osteotomy. Any residual discharge or secretion which might result from continuing otitis media, or indeed any portions of epithelial tissue inadvertently left behind, will accumulate and may well result in para-aural abscessation[3,26]. Most authorities recommend LBO in association with ablation of the external ear canal, since to perform ventral bulla osteotomy would require repositioning of the animal during surgery, an unnecessary complication since the ventral approach has no advantage over the lateral[29].

Presurgical evaluation of the facial, oculosympathetic, and vestibular (cranial nerve VIII) nerves is useful[28,30] as it provides a baseline for assessing the significance of any postoperative neurological signs. Bilateral total ear canal ablation (TECA) performed simultaneously has been reported to cause pharyngeal swelling[2], a complication of hypoglossal nerve damage. This complication may necessitate a tracheostomy to alleviate upper airway obstruction. For this reason some surgeons stage the procedure by allowing at least 2–3 weeks to lapse before performing a second TECA on a patient. However, other surgeons take the view that the advantages of a single episode of anaesthesia and a single period of postoperative pain outweigh the small risk of pharyngeal problems.

Total ablation and bulla osteotomy should render the ear deaf but, somewhat surprisingly, this does not always occur[31,32]. It is wise to try and assess the dog's auditory ability preoperatively and to demonstrate this to the owner[2] in an attempt to forestall unwarranted accusations of surgical ineptitude.

Systemic antibacterial therapy is indicated both pre- and postoperatively, beginning 7–14 days preoperatively[30]. The patient is anesthetized and the surgical area prepared as described above. The pinna is hung with atraumatic forceps and a full draping of the field is performed. A small rolled towel placed under the neck of the dog, to elevate the head to the level of the chest wall, facilitates exposure[2].

A circumferential incision is made around the acoustic meatus, severing the auricular cartilage but not penetrating the lateral skin surface of the pinna. The incision is continued to the level of the junction of the horizontal and vertical ear canals (Figure 8.18). It may be necessary to resect large areas of infected, hyperplastic tissue in some cases, with consequent implications for postoperative pinnal carriage.

Blunt dissection is used to expose the lateral surface of the vertical canal (Figure 8.19). The vertical canal is freed from the surrounding tissue using a combination of blunt and sharp dissection (Figures 8.20, 8.21). A dry gauze sponge can be helpful for bluntly rubbing the connective tissue from the vertical canal. Care should be taken to avoid haemorrhage from the rostral auricular artery and vein and from the auriculopalpebral (branch of the facial) and auriculotemporal (branch of the trigeminal) nerves in the cranial aspect of the dissection[30]. Damage to blood vessels in this area may lead to avascular necrosis of the pinna[2]. Haemorrhage may be controlled with electrocautery in the area around the vertical canal but not the horizontal canal; the risk to the facial nerve is too great[23].

Blunt dissection, keeping as close to the perichondrium as possible, is continued

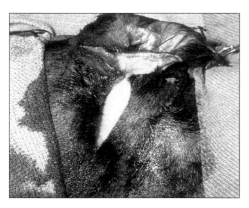

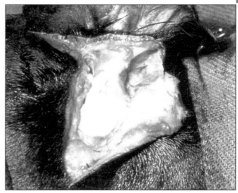

Fig. 8.18 Total ear canal ablation and bulla osteotomy. The initial incisions are made.

Fig. 8.19 The vertical ear canal is exposed, using blunt dissection.

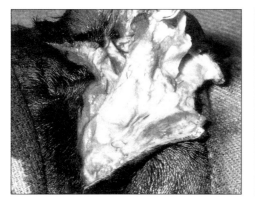

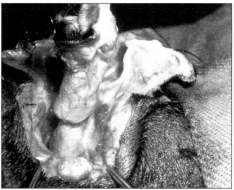

Figs. 8.20, 8.21 The external ear canal is gradually freed.

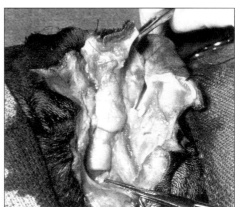

Fig. 8.22 Blunt dissection and gentle traction is used to enable the surgeon progressively to free the external ear canal to the level of the bony acoustic meatus.

around the angle that forms the transition between the vertical and horizontal canals, which represents the transition from auricular cartilage to annular cartilage (Figure 8.22). Care should be taken to identify the facial nerve as it exits from the stylomastoid foramen and curves rostroventrally around the horizontal

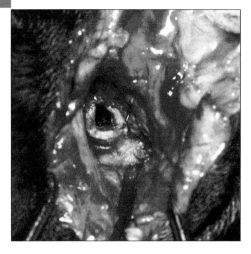

Fig. 8.23 The external ear canal is excised to expose the tympanic aperture.

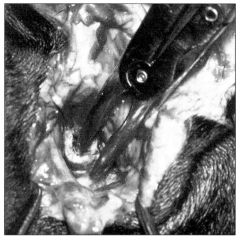

Fig. 8.24 Using rongeurs, the bony external acoustic meatus is removed to expose further the tympanic cavity.

canal. It should be carefully retracted ventrally. The advantage of performing this dissection after freeing the vertical canal is that there is maximal tissue laxity, which allows the fullest retraction[17]. In some cases the facial nerve may be intimately associated with perichondrial connective tissue or even buried within the reactive tissue surrounding ossified cartilage[1,26]. This will require careful dissection if significant postoperative morbidity is to be avoided. Gelpi retractors may be useful at this point. If the facial nerve proves hard to find, Smeak[17] advocated searching the caudal and more superficial aspect of the horizontal ear canal for small branches of the internal auricular nerve which penetrate the cartilage; these may be followed back to the facial nerve trunk. Gentle traction and tissue manipulation in this area is mandatory.

Blunt dissection is continued along the horizontal canal to the level of the skull. The entire horizontal canal is exposed to the level of the bony acoustic meatus, and then sharply transected, with scissors, at this level (Figure 8.23). If chronic disease has caused ossification of the horizontal canal, a small osteotome may be necessary to transect the ear canal. A clamp across the base of the horizontal canal before transection minimizes contamination from debris within the canal.

A bone curette is used to scrape all epithelial tissue from the osseous external acoustic meatus[27,30,33]. It is critical that all secretory tissue is removed as failure to achieve this will result in postoperative para-aural abscessation. The bony external acoustic meatus is removed (Figure 8.24) using a sharp, small rongeur (such as a Lempert rongeur) or an air drill. This will allow increased visualization of the tympanic cavity. When enlarging the external auditory meatus it is best to stay rostral and ventral to avoid the oval and round windows (on the opposite wall of the bulla to the tympanum) and the facial nerve[33].

The ventrolateral portion of the tympanic bulla is removed (Figure 8.25) with rongeurs or an air-driven burr. It may

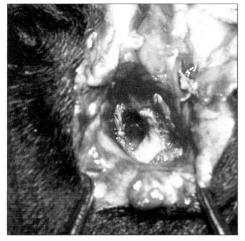

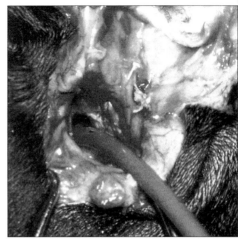

Fig. 8.25 The ventrolateral wall of the tympanic bulla has now been breached.

Fig. 8.26 After the tympanic cavity has been curetted it is flushed to ensure removal of all debris.

prove necessary to extend the osteotomy rostrally and caudally in order to visualize the caudal aspects of the tympanic cavity adequately. It is imperative that the shelf of bone ventromedial to the external acoustic meatus is removed if adequate exposure is to be achieved for optimum curettage[33].

The surgeon should avoid advancing onto the ventral aspect of the bulla. Some ventral retraction of the soft tissues will have been performed to allow dissection of the annular cartilage, but both the facial nerve and the external carotid artery are in this area and extreme caution is warranted. If haemorrhage is encountered, definitive haemostasis is important; use haemostatic clips[33].

Suction is usually necessary at this point to maintain adequate visibility of the surgical field. The tympanic cavity is curetted or abraded, using a dry gauze sponge wrapped on the end of a haemostat to remove any inspissated contents, secretory epithelium, and remnants of the tympanic membrane and the malleus, if not removed earlier. Care should be taken not to evulse the stapes off the oval window; peripheral vestibular problems may result. Paradoxically, removal of chronically inflamed epithelia is often more easily accomplished than removal of minimally inflamed tissue. Extreme care should be taken not to disrupt the epitympanic recess, the round window (mid-dorsal aspect), or the oval window (craniodorsal). Samples from the middle ear should be submitted for bacterial culture and sensitivity.

Note: This part of the procedure is critical, for if infected secretory tissue is left within the bulla, postoperative abscessation and fistulation can be expected.

The tympanic cavity is thoroughly flushed with warmed saline solution (Figure 8.26). A drain (latex, active, or ingress/egress) (Figure 8.27) may be placed, entering via the tympanic orifice and exiting the tympanic cavity through the osteotomy and passing through the skin via a stab incision. This is beneficial if clearing of the bulla is not complete or if a large amount of discharge is expected[2]. Drainage

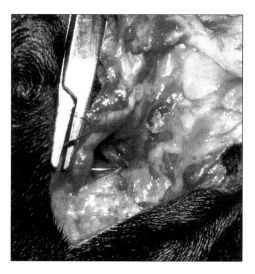

Fig. 8.27 A drain tube is placed (through a separate stab incision) and closure begun.

may not be necessary with strict adherence to good surgical techniques[34].

Closure is performed using monofilament absorbable sutures in the subcutaneous tissue (Figures 8.28–8.30). Great care must be taken to close all potential dead space as this will help to minimize postoperative cellulitis. Routine skin closure is performed in the shape of a 'T', with care taken to effect a cosmetic ear carriage when closing the area of the former tragus and antitragus.

Postsurgical care

Postoperative analgesia is mandatory. Postoperative systemic antibacterial therapy is usually warranted and must be continued for 10–21 days[2,30]. The choice of antibacterial agent may need to be reviewed in the light of bacterial culture and sensitivity testing of tissue obtained at surgery. Postoperative glucocorticoids have been recommended[23]. Used in anti-inflammatory doses (0.5–1.0 mg/kg divided q12 h) prednisolone may help to decrease postoperative swelling. Glucocorticoids should not be used for more than 3 days and care must

be taken to ensure that they are not used concurrently with nonsteroidal anti-inflammatory drugs as there is an increased risk of gastric ulceration.

Generally, it is not necessary to irrigate postoperatively; the drains are placed (Figures 8.31, 8.32) to allow local exudate to clear the surgical site rather than to facilitate flushing[30]. If a drain is inserted, soft, padded dressings should be used to cover the surgical site and the drain egress until the drain is removed, typically after 2–5 days. Care should be taken that these dressings do not constrict the pharynx[17]. Sutures are removed after 10–14 days.

Careful neurological observations should be made. In the immediate postoperative period, hypoglossal damage may be apparent and although it does not usually require specific treatment, animals should be closely observed for the 24 hours immediately postsurgery[2]. Respiratory function, in particular, should be monitored postoperatively as significant pharyngeal swelling may occur following bilateral surgery[17]. Ocular lubricants may be indicated until normal blink reflex is regained.

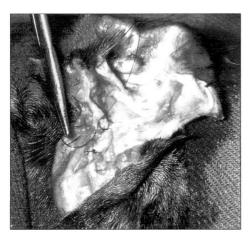
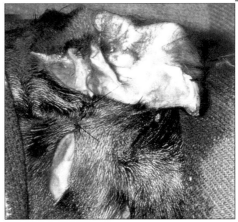
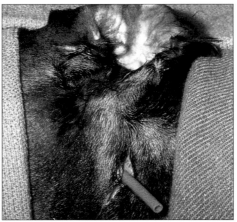

Figs. 8.28–8.30 Routine closure, ensuring elimination of dead space, ends the surgery.

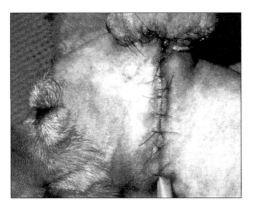
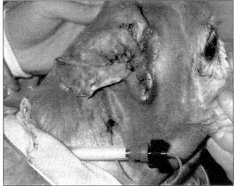

Figs. 8.31,8.32 Passive and active drains, put in place after surgery, ensure that any exudate is removed.

Postsurgical problems

Postsurgical problems are a reflection of two main factors: the surgical complexity of the procedure and the degree of bacterial contamination of the surgical site[2,21,35].

Discharge from the surgical site is common[2,26–28,33]. Discharge and post-operative swelling may be treated with hot compresses for 5 minutes, three times daily. Drainage may be facilitated by removing the most ventral sutures. Fistula formation (para-aural sinus) may occur 3–12 months postsurgery in cases in which incomplete removal of infected and secretory tissue was achieved. Para-aural sinuses (Figure 8.33) may create more clinical problems than the original otitis[17,35].

Pinnal necrosis (which is usually limited to the caudal aspect of the pinna) is a consequence of compromised blood supply. Management is based on local cleansing, debridement if necessary, and awaiting re-epithelialization.

Postoperative nerve damage is relatively common, and in about 10% of cases some degree of permanent neuropathy can be expected[2,27,30,34]. Hypoglossal nerve damage (drooling, dysphagia) is usually short term. Facial nerve damage is the most common

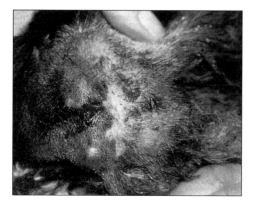

Fig. 8.33 Para-aural sinus following incomplete removal of all secretory tissues at surgery.

postoperative neuropathy[2,27,30,34]. Mild, transient paresis of the auriculopalpebral nerve is also common[21]. Ninety percent of these cases resolve within a few weeks of surgery and they can be managed by application of artificial tears, for example[35,36]. However, absence of blink reflex, lip paralysis, or pinnal paralysis may be long term, and the prognosis is poor if no evidence of improvement is apparent 4 weeks postsurgery[17]. The practical consequences of long-term facial nerve damage are minimal provided tear production is normal and exophthalmia is not present[17].

Postoperative Horner's syndrome and damage to the facial nerve (ptosis, midriasis, nystagmus, head tilt, flaccid facial paralysis) is usually confined to the cat and will resolve within a few weeks, as long as the otitis media has resolved[2].

Short-term complications, such as incisional abscess, dehiscence, or swelling, can be seen with TECA-LBO. Most are short lived and resolve with conservative treatment, although extensive complications may require surgical revision. If damage to the epitympanic recess, oval window, or round window occurs, abnormalities such as nystagmus, head tilt, and general vestibular abnormalities can occur. This complication is often temporary, and resolves within 7–10 days with only supportive care. If a patient displayed a head tilt prior to surgery, it will often persist in the acute postoperative period, with some patients remaining persistently abnormal.

Long-term complications usually involve abscessation of the middle ear and/or fistulation of tissues ventral to the middle ear. Most commonly this is due to incomplete excision of the membranous lining of the bulla[3,34]. Medical therapy of persistent or recurrent infection is rarely curative. Surgical re-exploration of the bulla to remove remaining epithelial tissue, combined with debridement of infected tissue and appropriate drainage, is used to control infection and this is effective in up to 85% of dogs with recurrent postoperative otitis[36,37].

Deafness and loss of hearing ability after total ablation and bulla osteotomy is a common concern of owners. Studies vary, but patients with severe proliferative canal disease tend to retain the same level of hearing they had prior to surgery, hence the value of preoperative assessment[31]. This also is true in most cases when comparing preoperative and postoperative brainstem auditory evoked responses[4,37].

BULLA OSTEOTOMY

Indications

The principle indication for bulla osteotomy is the treatment of refractory otitis media[29,30,33]. The procedure is most commonly performed in the dog in association with total ablation of the external ear canal, in which case a lateral bulla osteotomy is performed. The alternative approach to the bulla is a ventral approach, most often performed in the cat in the management of inflammatory polyps arising from the middle ear. Other, much less common, indications are the excision of neoplastic masses and the removal of cholesteatomas[17].

Surgical technique
Lateral bulla osteotomy as a separate procedure

LBO is more easily performed after TECA has been carried out, principally because of increased visualization[38]. The surgical technique is as follows (after Krahwinkel et al.[37], Barrett and Rathfon[39], and Boothe[40]):

- A skin incision is made over the external ear canal and extended ventrally beyond the level of the horizontal ear canal. The subcutaneous tissues are gently dissected to reveal the apposition of the parotid salivary gland and the horizontal ear canal.

- Gentle, ventral retraction of the parotid gland should reveal the facial nerve, which is carefully retracted caudoventrally to reveal the lateral aspect of the tympanic bulla.

- The bulla is further exposed using a periosteal elevator and broached with a Steinmann pin in a hand chuck. Care is needed here because the density of the bulla varies and is unpredictable; too much pressure and the pin may impact on the opposite side of the tympanic cavity. The pin enters on the caudolateral aspect of the bulla and is directed from a caudoventral direction so that if it impacts on the medial wall it avoids the mediodorsal wall.

- The osteotomy site is enlarged with rongeurs, observing the precautions outlined above.

- Samples for microbiological culture and sensitivity testing are taken and the tympanic cavity is flushed with warm isotonic saline until the run-out is clear of debris.

- If purulence is evident in the tympanic cavity, a drain tube is sometimes placed. This is sutured to adjacent soft tissues with 4/0 catgut and exited adjacent to the initial skin incision. Twice daily flushing with an appropriate antibacterial agent is performed until the drain is removed after 7 days. Flushing may not always be effective unless an ingress (dorsal via the tympanic opening)/egress (ventral) drain is used[26]. Passive ventral drainage may suffice in many cases.

Ventral bulla osteotomy

Ventral bulla osteotomy provides less opportunity for iatrogenic nerve damage, better visualization of the tympanic cavity, and more consistent ventral drainage than the lateral approach[41,42]. The reason that this approach is not used more frequently in dogs is that in most cases middle ear infection is associated with chronic external ear disease and both areas are then addressed in a unified field. Furthermore, in one study[29] there was little difference in postoperative complications compared with the lateral approach.

Ventral bulla osteotomy is the most frequently used approach in the cat, a reflection of otitis media occurring in the absence of chronic otitis externa in this species. Note that the bulla of the cat differs from that of the dog. The surgical technique is as follows (after Fossum[3], Harari[15], Smeak and de Hoff[26], Boothe[41], Seim[42], Denny[43], and McNutt and McCoy[44]):

- A sagittal incision is made immediately medial to the mandibular salivary gland, at a level midway between the angle of the mandible and the wings of the atlas (Figure 8.34). The thin myelohyoid muscle is split.
- The digastricus muscle is separated from the hyoglossal and styloglossal muscles by blunt dissection.
- The hypoglossal nerve and branches of the internal carotid artery are identified on the lateral aspect of the hyoglossal muscle and carefully retracted medially.
- Further retraction of the digastricus muscle (laterally) and of the hyoglossal muscle (medially) reveals the rounded bulge of the bulla between the jugular processes of the skull (caudal to the bulla) and the angular process of the mandible (rostral).

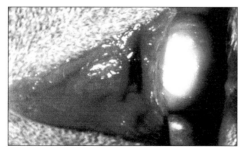

Fig. 8.34 The bulla has been exposed.

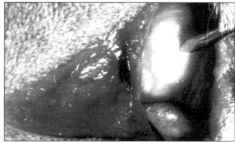

Fig. 8.35 A Steinmann pin has been used to broach the bulla.

- The thin muscular covering of the bulla is incised and reflected with a periosteal elevator.
- The bulla is broached with a Steinmann pin in a hand chuck (Figure 8.35). Care is needed here because sudden penetration may result in the pin impacting on the dorsal aspect of the tympanic cavity and damaging the oval or round windows.
- The pin is removed and the osteotomy site enlarged with rongeurs (Figures 8.36, 8.37).
- Samples for microbiological culture and sensitivity testing are taken and the tympanic cavity is flushed with warm isotonic saline until the run-out is clear of debris.

- A drain tube is placed if necessary (see above) in the tympanic cavity, sutured to adjacent soft tissues with 4/0 catgut, and exited adjacent to the initial skin incision. Twice daily flushing with an appropriate antibacterial agent is performed until drain removal after 7 days.

Postsurgical problems

Possible complications to bulla osteotomy are principally neurological[39]. As with those encountered after TECA and bulla osteotomy (described above), these relate principally to the hypoglossal nerve (drooling, dysphagia) and branches of the sympathetic and parasympathetic nerve supply (ipsilateral Horner's syndrome and keratoconjunctivitis sicca, respectively).

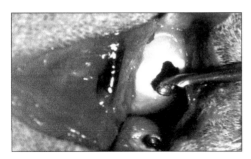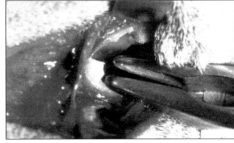

Figs. 8.36, 8.37 The osteotomy is progressively enlarged with rongeurs.

SPECIAL PROBLEMS RELATING TO SURGERY OF THE MIDDLE EAR IN CATS

Middle ear disease in cats usually relates to otitis media or inflammatory polyps, although neoplasia may occur rarely[45].

The tympanic bullae of cats are easily palpable on the ventral aspect of the feline skull and they are easily accessible with a straightforward dissection (Figure 8.38), as outlined above. However, the ventral chamber of the tympanic cavity is characterized by an incomplete bony septum[41]. It is this septum which is visible upon opening the ventral wall of the tympanic bulla and it divides the ventral cavity into two. The larger ventromedial chamber is entered via the bulla osteotomy and the smaller dorsolateral chamber, in effect the tympanic cavity proper, lies beyond the septum.

The two chambers communicate via the space between the septum and the caudomedial wall of the tympanic cavity[41]. The round window of the cochlea, the promontory, and the postganglionic fibres of the cervical sympathetic trunk are in this region of the medial wall and are thus vulnerable to damage, particularly if the septum is removed. Horner's syndrome will result if the sympathetic fibres are damaged. It may be necessary to open the septum if access to inflammatory polyps in the dorsolateral chamber is required or to facilitate drainage and, if so, care should be taken to avoid the region adjacent to the promontory[16]. Postoperative Horner's syndrome occurred in 42–57% of cases in one series[45,46]. Although the majority of cases resolved within 8 days of surgery, the signs persisted, albeit mildly, after 4 weeks in 21% of cases. Some facial paresis and inner ear disease (head tilt, ataxia) may also be noted postoperatively in a proportion of cases, again usually temporary[16].

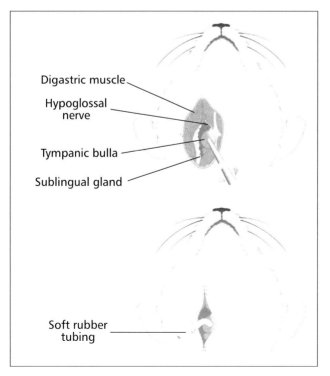

Fig. 8.38 Feline ventral bulla osteotomy. The surgical site.

Digastric muscle

Hypoglossal nerve

Tympanic bulla

Sublingual gland

Soft rubber tubing

CHAPTER 1 THE NORMAL EAR

Anatomy, structure and function

1 Getty R, Foust HL, Presley ET, Miller ME (1956). Macroscopic anatomy of the ear of the dog. *American Journal of Veterinary Research* **17**:364–375.

2 Fraser G, Gregor WW, Mackenzie CP, Spreull JSA, Withers AR (1970). Canine ear disease. *Journal of Small Animal Practice* **10**:725–754.

3 Evans HE (ed) (1993). *Miller's Anatomy of the Dog*, 3rd edn. WB Saunders, Philadelphia, pp. 988–1008.

4 Hudson LC, Hamilton WP (1993). *Atlas of Feline Anatomy for Veterinarians*. WB Saunders, Philadelphia, pp. 228–239.

5 Henderson RA, Horne RD (1993). The pinna. In: Slatter D (ed). *Textbook of Small Animal Surgery*, 2nd edn. WB Saunders, Philadelphia, pp. 1545–1559.

6 Smeak DD (1998). Total ear canal ablation and lateral bulla osteotomy. In: Bojrab MJ (ed). *Current Techniques in Small Animal Surgery*, 4th edn. Williams and Wilkins, Baltimore, pp. 102–109.

7 Huang H-P (1993). *Studies of the Microenvironment and Microflora of the Canine External Ear Canal*. PhD Thesis, Glasgow University.

8 Forsythe WB (1985). Tympanographic volume measurements of the canine ear. *American Journal of Veterinary Research* **46**:1351–1353.

9 Bluestone CD, Doyle WJ (1988). Anatomy and physiology of the eustachian tube and middle ear related to otitis media. *Journal of Allergy and Clinical Immunology* **81**:997–1003.

10 Bluestone CD (1983) Eustachian tube function: physiology, pathophysiology, and role of allergy in pathogenesis of otitis media. *Journal of Allergy and Clinical Immunology* **72**:242–251.

11 Ostfield E, Blonder J, Crispin M, Szeinberg A (1980). The middle ear gas composition in air-ventilated dogs. *Acta Otolaryngology* **89**:105–108.

12 Chole RA, Kodama K (1989). Comparative histology of the tympanic membrane and its relationship to cholesteatoma. *Annals of Rhinology and Laryngology* **98**:761–766.

13 Neer TM (1982). Otitis media. *Compendium on Continuing Education* **4**:410–416.

14 Nummela S (1995). Scaling of the mammalian middle ear. *Hearing Research* **85**:18–30.

15 Secondi U (1951). Structure and function of the lamina propria of the tympanic membrane in various mammals. *Archives of Otolaryngology* **53**:170–181.

16 Saridomichelakis MN, Farmaki R, Leontides LS, Koutinas AF (2007). Aetiology of canine otitis externa: a retrospective study of 100 cases. *Veterinary Dermatology* **18**:341–347.

Microscopic structure of the external ear canal

1 Fraser G (1961). The histopathology of the external auditory meatus of the dog. *Journal of Comparative Pathology* **71**:253–258.

2 Getty R, Foust HL, Presley ET, Miller ME (1956). Macroscopic anatomy of the ear of the dog. *American Journal of Veterinary Research* **17**:364–375.

3 Stout-Graham M, Kainer RA, Whalen LR, Macy DW (1990). Morphologic measurements of the external ear canal of dogs. *American Journal of Veterinary Research* **51**:990–994.

4 Huang H-P (1993). *Studies of the Microenvironment and Microflora of the Canine External Ear Canal*. PhD Thesis, Glasgow University.

5 Scott DW (1980). Feline dermatology: a monograph. *Journal of the American Animal Hospital Association* **16**:426–433.

6 Fernando SDA (1966). A histological and histochemical study of the glands of the external auditory canal of the dog. *Research in Veterinary Science* **7**:116–119.

7 Huang HP, Fixter LM, Little CJL (1994). Lipid content of cerumen from normal dogs and otitic canine ears. *Veterinary Record* **134**:380–381.

8 Fernando SDA (1966). A histological and histochemical study of the glands of the external auditory canal of the dog. *Research in Veterinary Science* **7**:116–119.

9 Huang HP, Little CJL (1994). Lipid content of cerumen from normal dogs and otitic canine ears. *Veterinary Record* **134**:380–381.

10 Huang HP, Little CJL, Fixter LM (1993). Effects of fatty acids on the growth and composition of *Malassezia pachydermatis* and their relevance to canine otitis externa. *Research in Veterinary Science* **55**:119–123.

11 Roeser RJ (1997). Physiology, pathophysiology, and anthropology / epidemiology of human ear canal secretions. *Journal of the American Academy of Audiology* **8**:391–400.

12 Gutteridge JMC, Lamport P, Dormandy TL (1974). Autoxidation as a cause of antibacterial activity in unsaturated fatty acids. *Journal of Medical Microbiology* **7**:387–389.

13 Knapp HR, Melly MA (1986). Bactericidal effects of polyunsaturated fatty acids. *Journal of Infectious Diseases* **154**:84–94.

14 Stout-Graham M, Kainer RA, Whalen LR, Macy DW (1990). Morphologic measurements of the external ear horizontal canal of dogs. *American Journal of Veterinary Research* **51**:990–994.

Microclimate of the external ear canal

1 Litton W (1963). Epithelial migration over the tympanum and external canal. *Archives of Otolaryngology* **77**:254–257.

2 Broekaert D (1990). The migratory capacity of the external auditory canal epithelium: a critical mini review. *Acta Oto-rhino-laryngologica (Belg)* **44**:385–392.

3 Grono LR (1970). Studies of the microclimate of the external auditory canal in the dog. 1: Aural temperature. *Research in Veterinary Science* **11**:307–311.

4 Huang H-P, Shih H-M, Chen K-Y (1998). The application of an infrared tympanic membrane thermometer in comparing the external ear canal temperature between erect and pendulous ears in dogs. In: Kwochka KW, Willemse T, von Tscharner C (eds). *Advances in Veterinary Dermatology*, Volume 3. Butterworth Heinemann, Oxford, pp. 57–63.

5 Hui-Pi Huang, Hui-Mei Shih (1998). Use of infrared thermometry and effect of otitis externa on external ear canal temperature in dogs. *Journal of the American Veterinary Medical Association* **213**:76–79.

6 Grono LR (1970). Studies of the microclimate of the external auditory canal in the dog. III: Relative humidity within the external auditory meatus. *Research in Veterinary Science* **11**:316–319.

7 Grono LR (1970). Studies of the microclimate of the external auditory canal in the dog. II: Hydrogen ion concentration of the external auditory meatus in the dog. *Research in Veterinary Science* **11**:312–315.

CHAPTER 2 APPROACH TO THE DIAGNOSIS OF OTITIS EXTERNA

Signalment

1 Saridomichelakis MN, Farmaki R, Leontides LS, Koutinas AF (2007). Aetiology of canine otitis externa: a retrospective study of 100 cases. *Veterinary Dermatology* **18**:341–347.

Otoscopic appearance of the external ear canal and tympanum

1 McKeever PJ, Richardson HW (1988). Otitis externa. Part 2: Clinical appearance and diagnostic methods. *Companion Animal Practice* **2**:25–31.

2 Getty R, Foust HL, Presley ET, Miller ME (1956). Macroscopic anatomy of the ear of the dog. *American Journal of Veterinary Research* **17**:364–375.

3 Stout-Graham M, Kainer RA, Whalen LR, Macy DW (1990). Morphologic measurements of the external ear canal of dogs. *American Journal of Veterinary Research* **51**:990–994.

4 Little CJL, Lane JG (1989). An evaluation of tympanometry, otoscopy and palpation for assessment of the canine tympanic membrane. *Veterinary Record* **124**:5–8.

5 Fraser G, Gregor WW, Mackenzie CP, Spreull JSA, Withers AR (1970). Canine ear disease. *Journal of Small Animal Practice* **10**:725–754.

6 Neer TM (1982). Otitis media. *Compendium on Continuing Education* **4**:410–416.

7 Fraser G (1965). Aetiology of otitis externa in the dog. *Journal of Small Animal Practice* **6**:445–452.

8 Huang HP, Fixter LM, Little CJL (1994). Lipid content of cerumen from normal dogs and otitic canine ears. *Veterinary Record* **134**:380–381.

Cytological characteristics of normal and abnormal ears

1 Griffin CE (1993). Otitis externa and otitis media. In: Griffin CE, Kwochka KW, MacDonald JM (eds). *Current Veterinary Dermatology*. Mosby, St Louis, pp. 245–262.

2 Rosser EJ (1988). Evaluation of the patient with otitis externa. *Veterinary Clinics of North America* **18**:765–772.

3 Huang H-P (1993). *Studies of the Microenvironment and Microflora of the Canine External Ear Canal*. PhD Thesis, Glasgow University.

4 Kowalski JJ (1988). The microbial environment of the ear canal in health and disease. *Veterinary Clinics of North America* **18**:743–754.

5 Chickering WR (1988). Cytologic evaluation of otic exudates. *Veterinary Clinics of North America* **18**:773–782.

6 Lehner G, Louis CS, Mueller RS (2010). Reproducibilty of ear cytology in dogs with otitis externa. *Veterinary Record* **167**:23–26.

7 Bouassiba C, Osthold W, Mueller RS (2013). Comparison of four different staining methods for ear cytology of dogs with otitis externa. *Tierarztliche Praxis Ausgabe Kleintiere Heimtiere* **41**:7–15.

8 Rosychuck RWA (1994). Management of otitis externa. *Veterinary Clinics of North America* **24**:921–952.

9 Huang H-P (1995). Canine cerumen cytology. *Chinese Society of Veterinary Science* **21**:18–23.

10 Huang H-P, Little CJL (1994). Lipid content of cerumen from normal dogs and otitic canine ears. *Veterinary Record* **134**:380–381.

11 Mansfield PD, Boosinger TR, Attleburger MH (1990). Infectivity of *Malassezia pachydermatis* in the external ear canal of dogs. *Journal of the American Animal Hospital Association* **26**:97–100.

12 Bond R, Anthony RM, Dodd M, Lloyd DH (1996). Isolation of *Malassezia sympodialis* from feline skin. *Journal of Medical and Veterinary Mycology* **34**:145–147.

13 Frost CR (1961). Canine otocariasis. *Journal of Small Animal Practice* **2**:253–256.

Video-otoscopic examination of the ear canal

1 Angus JC, Campbell KL (2001). Uses and indications for video-otoscopy in small animal practice. *Veterinary Clinics of North America Small Animal Practice* **31**:809–828.

2 Cole LK (2004). Otoscopic evaluation of the ear canal. *Veterinary Clinics of North America Small Animal Practice* **34**:397–410.

3 Usui R, Usui R, Fukuda M, Fukui E, Hasegawa A (2011). Treatment of canine otitis externa using video otoscopy. *Journal of Veterinary Medicine and Science* **73**:1249–1253.

Virtual otoscopy for evaluating the inner ear

1 Cho Y, Jeong J, Lee H, Kim, M, Kim N, Lee K (2012). Virtual otoscopy for evaluating the inner ear with a fluid filled tympanic cavity in dogs. *Journal of Veterinary Science* **14**:419–424.

2 Eom K, Kwak H, Kang H, *et al.* (2008). Virtual CT otoscopy of the middle ear and ossicles in dogs. *Veterinary Radiology and Ultrasound* **49**:545–550.

Radiography

1 Hare WCD (1958). Radiographic anatomy of the canine skull. *Journal of the American Veterinary Medical Association* **133**:149–157.

2 Gibbs C (1978). Radiological refresher. Part III. The head. *Journal of Small Animal Practice* **19**:539–545.

3 Rose WR (1977). Small animal clinical otology: radiology. *Veterinary Medicine/ Small Animal Clinician* **72**:1508–1517.

4 Love NE, Kramer RW, Spodnick GJ, Thrall DE (1995). Radiographic and computed tomographic evaluation of otitis media. *Veterinary Radiology and Ultrasound* **36**:375–379.

5 Douglas SW, Herrtage ME, Williamson HD (1987). Canine radiography: skull. In: *Principles of Veterinary Radiography*. Bailliére Tindall, London, pp. 177–192.

6 Sullivan M (1995). The head and neck. In: Lee R (ed). *BSAVA Manual of Small Animal Diagnostic Imaging*. British Small Animal Veterinary Association, Cheltenham, pp. 16–22.

7 Hoskinson JJ (1993). Imaging techniques in the diagnosis of middle ear disease. *Seminars in Veterinary Medicine* **8**:10–16.

8 Smeak DD, Kerpsack SJ (1993). Total ear canal ablation and lateral bulla osteotomy for management of end-stage otitis. *Seminars in Veterinary Medicine* **8**:30–41.

9 Remedios AM, Fowler JD, Pharr JW (1991). A comparison of radiographic versus surgical diagnosis of otitis media. *Journal of the American Animal Hospital Association* **27**:183–188.

10 Kealy JK (1987). The skull and vertebral column. In: Kealy JK (ed). *Diagnostic Radiology of the Dog and Cat*, 2nd edn. WB Saunders, Philadelphia, pp. 439–441.

11 Rohleder JJ, Jones JC, Duncan RB, Larsson MM, Waldron DL, Tromblee T (2006). Comparative performance of radiology and computed tomography in the diagnosis of middle ear disease in 31 dogs. *Veterinary Radiology and Ultrasound* **47**:45–52.

12 Doust R, King A, Hammond G, Cave T, Weinrauch S, Mellor D, Sullivan M (2007). Assessment of middle ear disease in the dog: a comparison of diagnostic imaging modalities. *Journal of Small Animal Practice* **48**:188–192.

13 King AM, Weinrauch SA, Doust R, Hammond G, Yam PS, Sullivan M (2007). Comparison of ultrasonography, radiology, and a single computed tomography slice for fluid identification within feline tympanic bulla. *Veterinary Journal* **173**:638–644.

14 Trower ND, Gregory SP, Renfrew H, Lamb CR (1998). Evaluation of canine tympanic membrane by positive contrast ear canalography. *Veterinary Record* **142**:78–81.

15 Eom K-D, Lee H-C, Yoon Y-H (2000). Canalographic evaluation of the external ear canal in dogs. *Veterinary Radiology and Ultrasound* **41**:231–234.

CHAPTER 3 AETIOLOGY AND PATHOGENESIS OF OTITIS EXTERNA

Concept of primary and secondary factors, predisposing factors, and perpetuating change

1 August JR (1988). Otitis externa. A disease of multifactorial etiology. *Veterinary Clinics of North America* **18**:731–742.

2 Griffin CE (2010). Classifying cases of otitis externa the PSPP System. *Proceedings of ESVD Workshop of Otitis*, St Helens.

Hypersensitivities

1 Halliwell REW, Gorman NT (1989). Atopic disease. In: Halliwell REW, Gorman NT (eds). *Veterinary Clinical Immunology*. WB Saunders, Philadelphia, pp. 232–252.
2 Scott DW (1981). Observations on canine atopy. *Journal of the American Animal Hospital Association* **17**:91–100.
3 Griffin CE (1993). Canine atopic disease. In: Griffin CE, Kwochka KW, MacDonald JM (eds). *Current Veterinary Dermatology*, Mosby, St Louis, pp. 99–120.
4 Harvey RG (1993). Food allergy and dietary intolerance in dogs: a report of 25 cases. *Journal of Small Animal Practice* **34**:175–179.
5 Rosser EJ (1993). Diagnosis of food allergy in dogs. *Journal of the American Veterinary Medical Association* **203**:259–262.
6 Carlotti DN, Remy I, Prost C (1990). Food allergy in dogs and cats: a review and report of 43 cases. *Veterinary Dermatology* **1**:55–62.
7 White SD, Sequoia D (1989). Food hypersensitivity in cats: 14 cases (1982–1987). *Journal of the American Veterinary Medical Association* **194**:692–695.
8 Walder EJ, Conroy JD (1994). Contact dermatitis in dogs and cats: pathogenesis, histopathology, experimental induction, and case reports. *Veterinary Dermatology* **5**:149–162.
9 Nesbitt GH, Schmitz JA (1977). Contact dermatitis in the dog: a review of 35 cases. *Journal of the American Animal Hospital Association* **13**:155–163.
10 Griffin CE (1993). Otitis externa and otitis media. In: Griffin CE, Kwochka KW, MacDonald JM (eds). *Current Veterinary Dermatology*, Mosby, St Louis, pp. 245–262.

Autoimmune/immune mediated

1 Scott DW, Miller WJ Jnr, Lewis RM, Manning TO, Smith CA (1980). Pemphigus erythematosus in the dog and cat. *Journal of the American Animal Hospital Association* **16**:815–823.
2 Manning TO, Scott DW, Smith CA, Lewis RM (1982). Pemphigus diseases in the feline: seven case reports and discussion. *Journal of the American Animal Hospital Association* **18**:433–443.
3 Scott DW, Walton DK, Manning TO, Smith CA, Lewis RM (1983). Canine lupus erythematosus. 1: Systemic lupus erythematosus. *Journal of the American Animal Hospital Association* **19**:561–579.
4 Ihrke PJ, Stannard AA, Ardans AA, Griffin CE (1985). Pemphigus foliaceus in dogs: a review of 37 cases. *Journal of the American Veterinary Medical Association* **186**:59–66.

Ectoparasitic causes

1 Scott DW, Horn RT (1987). Zoonotic dermatoses of dogs and cats. *Veterinary Clinics of North America* **17**:117–144.
2 Powell MB, Weisbroth SH, Roth L, Wilhelmsen C (1980). Reaginic hypersensitivity in Otodectes cynotis infestation of cats and mode of mite feeding. *American Journal of Veterinary Research* **6**:877–881.
3 Larkin AD, Gaillard GE (1981). Mites in cats' ears: a source of cross antigenicity with house dust mites. *Annals of Allergy* **46**:301–304.
4 Kuwahara J (1986). Canine and feline aural hematoma: clinical, experimental, and clinicopathologic observations. *American Journal of Veterinary Research* **47**:2300–2308.
5 Kuwahara J (1986). Canine and feline aural hematomas: results of treatment with corticosteroids. *Journal of the American Animal Hospital Association* **22**:641–647.
6 Hewitt M, Walton GS, Waterhouse M (1971). Pet animal infestations and skin lesions. *British Journal of Dermatology* **85**:215–255.
7 Frost CR (1961). Canine otocariasis. *Journal of Small Animal Practice* **2**:253–256.
8 Scott DW (1980). Feline dermatology 1900–1978. A monograph. *Journal of the American Animal Hospital Association* **16**:331–459.

9   Park G-S, Park J-S, Cho B-K, Lee W-K, Cho J-H (1996). Mite infestation rate of pet dogs with ear dermatoses. *Korean Journal of Parasitology* **34**:143–150.

10   Grono LR (1969). Studies of the ear mite, *Otodectes cynotis*. *Veterinary Record* **85**:6–8.

11   Knottenbelt MK (1994). Chronic otitis externa due to *Demodex canis* in a Tibetan Spaniel. *Veterinary Record* **135**:409–410.

12   Greene RT, Scheidt VJ and Moncol DJ (1986) Trombiculiasis in a cat. *Journal of the American Veterinary Medical Association* **188**:1054–1055.

13   Moriello KA (1987). Common ectoparasites of the dog. Part 1: Fleas and ticks. *Canine Practice* **14**:6–18.

14   White SD, Scott KV, Cheney JM (1995). *Otobius megnini* infestation in three dogs. *Veterinary Dermatology* **6**:33–35.

Endocrinopathies

1   Pancierra DL (1994). Hypothyroidism in dogs: 66 cases (1987–1992). *Journal of the American Veterinary Medical Association* **204**:761–767.

2   Ling GV, Stabenfeldt GH, Comer KM, Gribble DH, Schechter RD (1979). Canine hyperadrenocorticism: pretreatment clinical and laboratory evaluation of 117 cases. *Journal of the American Veterinary Medical Association* **174**:1211–1215.

3   White SD, Ceragioli KL, Bullock LP, Mason GD (1989). Cutaneous markers of canine hyperadrenocorticism. *Compendium on Continuing Education* **11**:446–464.

4   Schmeitzel LP, Lothrop CD (1990). Sex hormones and the skin. *Veterinary Medicine Report* **2**:28–41.

Epithelialization disorders

1   Paradis M, Scott DW (1990). Hereditary primary seborrhoea in Persian cats. *Feline Practice* **18**:17–20.

2   Kwochka KW (1993). Overview of normal keratinization and cutaneous scaling disorders of dogs. In: Griffin CE, Kwochka KW, MacDonald JM (eds). *Current Veterinary Dermatology*, Mosby, St Louis, pp. 167–175.

3   Kwochka KW, Rademakers AM (1989). Cell proliferation kinetics of epidermis, hair follicles, and sebaceous glands of Cocker Spaniels with idiopathic seborrhea. *American Journal of Veterinary Research* **50**:1918–1922.

4   Scott DW, Miller WH Jnr (1989). Epidermal dysplasia and *Malassezia pachydermatis* infection in West Highland White Terriers. *Veterinary Dermatology* **1**:25–36.

5   Maudlin EA, Scott DW, Miller WH Jnr, Smith CA (1997). *Malassezia* dermatitis in the dog: a retrospective histopathological and immunopathological study of 86 cases (1990–95). *Veterinary Dermatology* **8**:183–190.

6   Bond R, Rose JF, Ellis JW, Lloyd DH (1995). Comparison of two shampoos for treatment of *Malassezia pachydermatis*-associated seborrhoeic dermatitis in Basset Hounds. *Journal of Small Animal Practice* **36**:99–104.

Foreign bodies

1   McKeever PJ, Torres S (1988). Otitis externa. Part 1: The ear and predisposing factors to otitis externa. *Companion Animal Practice* **2**:7–14.

2   Brennan KE, Ihrke PJ (1983). Grass awn migration in dogs and cats: a retrospective study of 182 cases. *Journal of the American Veterinary Medical Association* **182**:1201–1204.

3   Rycroft AK, Saben HS (1977). A clinical study of otitis externa in the dog. *Canadian Veterinary Journal* **18**:64–70.

4   Roth L (1988). Pathologic changes in otitis externa. *Veterinary Clinics of North America* **14**:755–764.

Microbiological changes associated with otitis externa

1   Fraser G (1961). Factors predisposing to canine external otitis. *Veterinary Record* **73**:55–58.

2   McCarthy G and Kelly WR (1982). Microbial species associated with the canine ear and their antibacterial sensitivity patterns. *Irish Veterinary Journal* **36**:53–56.

3 Uchida Y, Tetsuya N, Kitazawa K (1990). Clinicomicrobiological study of the normal and otitis externa ear canals in dogs and cats. *Japanese Journal of Veterinary Science* **52**:415–417.

4 Gustafson B (1954). Otitis externa hos hund. *Nordic Veterinærmedicin* **6**:434–44.

5 Grono LR, Frost AJ (1969). Otitis externa in the dog. *Australian Veterinary Journal* **45**:420–422.

6 Sharma VD, Rhodes HE (1975). The occurrence and microbiology of otitis externa in the dog. *Journal of Small Animal Practice* **16**:241–247.

7 Chengappa MM, Maddux R, Greer S (1983). A microbiologic survey of clinically normal and otitic ear canals. *Pet Practice* **78**:343–344.

8 Marshall MJ, Harris AM, Horne JE (1974). The bacteriological and clinical assessment of a new preparation for the treatment of otitis externa in dogs and cats. *Journal of Small Animal Practice* **15**:401–410.

9 McKellar QA, Rycroft A, Anderson L, Love J (1990). Otitis externa in a foxhound pack associated with *Candida albicans*. *Veterinary Record* **127**:15–16.

10 Fraser G (1961). The fungal flora of the canine ear. *Journal of Comparative Pathology* **71**:1–5.

11 Fraser G, Withers AR, Spreull JSA (1961). Otitis externa in the dog. *Journal of Small Animal Practice* **2**:32–47.

12 Baxter M, Lawler DC (1972). The incidence and microbiology of otitis externa of dogs and cats in New Zealand. *New Zealand Veterinary Journal* **20**:29–32.

13 Krogh HV, Linnel A, Knudsen PB (1975). Otitis externa in the dog: a clinical and microbiological study. *Nordic Veterinærmedicin* **27**:285–295.

14 Baba E, Fukata T, Saito M (1981). Incidence of otitis externa in dogs and cats in Japan. *Veterinary Record* **108**:393–395.

15 Blue JL, Wooley RE (1977). Antibacterial sensitivity patterns of bacteria isolated from dogs with otitis externa. *Journal of the American Veterinary Medical Association* **171**:362–363.

16 Nesbitt GH, Schmitz JA (1977). Chronic bacterial dermatitis and otitis: a review of 195 cases. *Journal of the American Animal Hospital Association* **13**:442–450.

17 Webster FL, Whyard BH, Brandt RW, Jones WG (1974). Treatment of otitis externa in the dog with Gentocin Otic. *Canadian Veterinary Journal* **15**:176–177.

18 Rycroft AK, Saban HS (1977). A clinical study of otitis externa in the dog. *Canadian Veterinary Journal* **18**:64–70.

19 Oliveira LC, Leite CAL, Brihante RSN, Carvalho CBM (2009). Comparative study of the microbial profile from bilateral canine otitis externa. *Canadian Veterinary Journal* **49**:785–788.

20 Hallu RE, Gentilini E, Rebuelto M, Albarellos GA, Otero PE (1996). The combination of norfloxacin and ketoconazole in the treatment of canine otitis. *Canine Practice* **21**:26–28.

21 Fraser G (1961). The fungal flora of the canine ear. *Journal of Comparative Pathology* **71**:1–5.

Response to insult and injury

1 Fernando SDA (1966). Certain histopathological features of the external auditory meatus of the cat and dog with otitis externa. *American Journal of Veterinary Research* **28**:278–282.

2 van der Gagg I (1986). The pathology of the external ear canal in dogs and cats. *Veterinary Quarterly* **8**:307–317.

3 Fraser G (1961). The histopathology of the external auditory meatus of the dog. *Journal of Comparative Pathology* **71**:253–258.

4 Stout-Graham M, Kainer RA, Whalen LR, Macy DW (1990). Morphologic measurements of the external ear canal of dogs. *American Journal of Veterinary Research* **51**:990–994.

5 Huang HP, Fixter LM, Little CJL (1994). Lipid content of cerumen from normal dogs and otitic canine ears. *Veterinary Record* **134**:380–381.

6 Grono LR (1970). Studies of the microclimate of the external auditory canal in the dog. III: Relative humidity within the external auditory meatus. *Research in Veterinary Science* **11**:316–319.

7 Fraser G, Gregor WW, Mackenzie CP, Spreull JSA, Withers AR (1970). Canine ear disease. *Journal of Small Animal Practice* **10**:725–754.

8 Lane JG, Little CJL (1986). Surgery of the external auditory meatus: a review of failures. *Journal of Small Animal Practice* **27**:247–254.

Influence of breed

1 Fernando SDA (1966). A histological and histochemical study of the glands of the external auditory canal of the dog. *Research in Veterinary Science* **7**:116–119.

2 Stout-Graham M, Kainer RA, Whalen LR, Macy DW (1990). Morphologic measurements of the external ear canal of dogs. *American Journal of Veterinary Research* **51**:990–994.

3 Baxter M, Lawler DC (1972). The incidence and microbiology of otitis externa of dogs and cats in New Zealand. *New Zealand Veterinary Journal* **20**:29–32.

4 Hayes HM, Pickle LW, Wilson GP (1987). Effects of ear type and weather on the prevalence of canine otitis externa. *Research in Veterinary Science* **42**:294–298.

5 Fraser G (1965). Aetiology of otitis externa in the dog. *Journal of Small Animal Practice* **6**:445–452.

6 Fraser G (1961). The fungal flora of the canine ear. *Journal of Comparative Pathology* **71**:1–5.

7 Fraser G, Withers AR, Spreull JSA (1961). Otitis externa in the dog. *Journal of Small Animal Practice* **2**:32–47.

8 Krogh HV, Linnel A, Knudsen PB (1975). Otitis externa in the dog: a clinical and microbiological study. *Nordic Veterinærmedicin* **27**:285–295.

9 Baba E, Fukata T, Saito M (1981). Incidence of otitis externa in dogs and cats in Japan. *Veterinary Record* **108**:393–395.

Excessive moisture

1 Grono LR (1970). Studies of the microclimate of the external auditory canal in the dog. I: Aural temperature. *Research in Veterinary Science* **11**:307–311.

2 Grono LR (1970). Studies of the microclimate of the external auditory canal in the dog. III: Relative humidity within the external ear auditory meatus. *Research in Veterinary Science* **11**:316–319.

3 Hayes HM, Pickle LW, Wilson GP (1987). Effects of ear type and weather on the prevalence of canine otitis externa. *Research in Veterinary Science* **42**:294–298.

4 Grono LR, Frost AJ (1969). Otitis externa in the dog. *Australian Veterinary Journal* **45**:420–422.

5 Wilkinson JD (1992). The external ear. In: Champion RH, Burton JL, Ebling FJG (eds). *Textbook of Dermatology*, 4th edn. Blackwell Scientific Publications, Oxford, pp. 2671–2688.

6 Pack GE, Ayres JG (1985). Asthma outbreaks during a thunderstorm. *Lancet* **2**:199–203.

7 Knox RB (1993). Grass pollen, thunderstorms and asthma. *Clinical and Experimental Allergy* **23**:345–359.

Obstructive disease

1 London CA, Dubilzieg RR, Vail DM, *et al.* (1996). Evaluation of dogs and cats with tumors of the ear canal: 145 cases (1978–1992). *Journal of the American Veterinary Medical Association* **208**:1413–1418.

2 van der Gaag I (1986). The pathology of the external ear canal in dogs and cats. *Veterinary Quarterly* **8**:307–317.

3 Legendre AM, Krahwinkel AJ (1981). Feline ear tumours. *Journal of the American Animal Hospital Association* **17**:1035–1037.

4 Goldschmidt MH, Shofer FS (1992). Ceruminous gland tumors. In: Goldschmidt MH, Shofer FS (eds). *Skin Tumors of the Dog and Cat*. Pergamon Press, New York, pp. 96–102.

5 Kirpenstein J (1993). Aural neoplasms. *Seminars in Veterinary Medicine and Surgery (Small Animal)* **8**:17–23.

6 Goldschmidt MH, Shofer FS (1992). Cutaneous fibrosarcoma. In: Goldschmidt MH, Shofer FS (eds). *Skin Tumors of the Dog and Cat*. Pergamon Press, New York, pp. 158–167.

7 Marino DJ, MacDonald JM, Matthiesen DT, Patnaik AK (1994). Results of surgery in cats with ceruminous gland adenocarcinoma. *Journal of the American Animal Hospital Association* **30**:54–58.

8 Marino DJ, MacDonald JM, Matthiesen DT, Salmeri KR, Patnaik AK (1993). Results of surgery and long-term follow-up in dogs with ceruminous gland adenocarcinoma. *Journal of the American Animal Hospital Association* **29**:560–563.

9 Theon AP, Barthez PY, Madewell BR, Griffey SM (1994). Radiation therapy of ceruminous gland carcinomas in dogs and cats. *Journal of the American Veterinary Medical Association* **205**:566–569.

10 Howlett CR, Allan GS (1974). Tumours of the feline ear canal. *Australian Veterinary Practitioner* **4**:56–57.

11 Poulet FM, Valentine BA, Scott DW (1991). Focal proliferative eosinophilic dermatitis of the external ear canal in four dogs. *Veterinary Pathology* **28**:171–173.

CHAPTER 4 EAR CLEANING

1 Little CJ (1996). Medical treatment of otitis externa in the dog and cat. *In Practice* **18**:66–71.

2 McKeever PJ (1996). Otitis externa. *Compendium on Continuing Education* **18**:759–772.

3 Mansfield PD, Steiss JE, Boosinger TR, Marshall AE (1997). The effect of four commercially available ceruminolytic agents on the middle ear. *Journal of the American Animal Hospital Association* **33**:479–486.

4 Griffin CE (1993). Otitis externa and otitis media. In: Griffin CE, Kwochka KW, MacDonald JM (eds). *Current Veterinary Dermatology*. CE Mosby, St Louis, pp. 245–262.

5 Robinson AC, Hawke M, Mackay A, Ekem JK, Stratis M (1989). The mechanism of ceruminolysis. *Journal of Otolaryngology* **18**:268–273.

6 McKeever PJ, Richardson HW (1988). Otitis externa. Part 3: Ear cleaning and medical treatment. *Companion Animal Practice* **2**:24–30.

7 Rosychuck RAW (1994). Management of otitis externa. *Veterinary Clinics of North America* **24**:921–952.

8 Chester DK (1988). Medical management of otitis externa. *Veterinary Clinics of North America* **18**:799–812.

9 Robinson AC, Hawke M (1989). The efficacy of ceruminolytics: everything old is new again. *Journal of Otolaryngology* **18**:263–267.

10 Bruyette DS, Lorenz MD (1993). Otitis externa and otitis media: diagnostic and medical aspects. *Seminars in Veterinary Medicine and Surgery (Small Animal)* **8**:3–9.

11 Wilcke JR (1988). Otopharmacology. *Veterinary Clinics of North America* **18**:783–798.

12 Merchant SR, Neer TM, Tedford BL, Tewdt AC, Cheramie OM, Strain GM (1995). Ototoxicity of a chlorhexidine otic preparation in dogs. *Progress in Veterinary Neurology* **4**:72–75.

13 Igashi Y, Oka Y (1988). Vestibular ototoxicity following intratympanic application of chlorhexidine gluconate in the cat. *Archives of Otorhinolaryngology* **245**:210–217.

14 Jaffray B, King PM, Macleod DA, Wiseman R (1990). Bacterial colonisation of the skin after chemical depilation. *Journal of the Royal College of Surgeons (Edinburgh)* **35**:243–244.

15 Sanchez IR, Swaim SF, Nusbaum KE, Hale AS, Henderson RA, McGuire JA (1988). Effects of chlorhexidine diacetate and povidine-iodine on wound healing in dogs. *Veterinary Surgery* **17**:291–295.

16 Lee AH, Swaim SF, McGuire JA, Hughes KS (1988). Effects of chlorhexidine diacetate, povidine iodine and polyhydroxydine on wound healing in dogs. *Journal of the American Animal Hospital Association* **24**:77–84.

17   Rackur H (1985). New aspects of mechanism of action of povidine-iodine. *Journal of Hospital Infection* **6**:13–23.

18   Steen SI, Paterson S (2012). The susceptibility of *Pseudomonas* spp. isolated from dogs with otitis to topical ear cleaners. *Journal of Small Animal Practice* **53**:599–603.

19   Lineaweaver W, McMorris S, Soucy D, Howard R (1985). Cellular and bacterial toxicities of topical antimicrobials. *Plastic and Reconstructive Surgery* **75**:394–396.

20   Swinney A, Fazakerley J, McEwan N, Nuttall T (2008). Comparative *in vitro* antimicrobial efficacy of commercial ear cleaners. *Veterinary Dermatology* **19**:373–379.

21   Guardabassi L, Giovanni G, Damborg P (2010). *In vitro* antimicrobial activity of a commercial ear antiseptic containing chlorhexidine and Tris–EDTA. *Veterinary Dermatology* **21**:282–286.

22   Farca AM, Nebbia P, Re G (1991). Potentiation of the *in vitro* activity of some antimicrobial agents against selected Gram negative bacteria by EDTA tromethamine. *Veterinary Research Communications* **17**:77–84.

23   Cole LK, Kwochka KW, Kowalski JJ, Hillier A (2003). Evaluation of an ear cleanser for the treatment of infectious otitis externa in dogs. *Veterinary Theraputics* **4**:12–23.

24   Lloyd DH, Lamport AI (2000). Evaluation *in vitro* of the antimicrobial activity of two topical preparations used in the management of ear infections in the dog. *Veterinary Therepeutics* **1**:43–47.

25   Reme CA, Pin D, Collinot C, Cadiergues MC, Joyce JA, Fontaine J (2006). The efficacy of an antiseptic and microbial anti-adhesive ear cleanser in dogs with otitis externa. *Veterinary Therapeutics* **7**:15–26.

26   Gotthelf LN (2005). Ototoxicity. In: Gotthelf LN (ed). *Small Animal Ear Diseases: An Illustrated Guide*, 2nd edn. Elsevier Saunders, St Louis, pp. 329–337.

CHAPTER 5 MEDICAL MANAGEMENT OF EAR DISEASE

1   Scott DW, Horn RT (1987). Zoonotic dermatoses of dogs and cats. *Veterinary Clinics of North America* **17**:117–144.

2   Powell MB, Weisbroth SH, Roth L, Wilhelmsen C (1980). Reaginic hypersensitivity in *Otodectes cynotis* infestation of cats and mode of mite feeding. *American Journal of Veterinary Research* **6**:877–881.

3   Clayton TM (1943). Treatment of scabies by T.E.T.S. *British Medical Journal* **1**:443–445.

4   Gold S (1966). A skin full of alcohol. *Lancet* **ii**:1417.

5   Evans JM, Jemmett JE (1978). Otitis externa: the case for polypharmacy. *New Zealand Veterinary Journal* **26**:280–283.

6   Hewitt M, Walton GS, Waterhouse M (1971). Pet infestations and skin lesions. *British Journal of Dermatology* **85**:215–255.

7   Chester DK (1988). Medical management of otitis externa. *Veterinary Clinics of North America* **18**:799–812.

8   Scott DW (1980). Feline dermatology 1900–1978. A monograph. *Journal of the American Animal Hospital Association* **16**:331–459.

9   White SD, Scott KV, Cheney JM (1995). *Otobius megnini* infestation in three dogs. *Veterinary Dermatology* **6**:33–35.

10   Hansen SR (1995). Management of adverse reactions to pyrethrins and pyrethroid insecticides. In: Bonagura JD (ed). *Current Veterinary Therapy XII*. WB Saunders, Philadelphia, pp. 242–245.

11   Hansen SR (1995). Management of organophosphate and carbamate toxicoses. In: Bonagura JD (ed). *Current Veterinary Therapy XII*. WB Saunders, Philadelphia, pp. 245–248.

12   Mueller RD, Bettenay SV (1999). A proposed new therapeutic protocol for the treatment of canine mange with ivermectin. *Journal of the American Animal Hospital Association* **35**:77–80.

13   Schneck G (1988). Use of ivermectin against ear mites in cats. *Veterinary Record* **123**:599.

14 Gram D (1991). Treatment of ear mites (*Otodectes cynotis*) in cats: comparison of subcutaneous and topical ivermectin. *Proceedings 7th Annual Meeting AAVD/ACVD*, Scottsdale, p 26.

15 Paradis M (1998). Ivermectin in small animal dermatology. Part 1: Pharmacology and toxicology. *Compendium on Continuing Education* **20**:193–199.

16 Dorman DC (1995). Neurotoxic drugs in dogs and cats. In: Bonagura JD (ed). *Current Veterinary Therapy XII*. WB Saunders, Philadelphia, pp. 1140–1145.

17 Paul AJ, Tranquilli WJ, Seward RL, Todd KS Jnr, DiPietro JA (1987). Clinical observations in Collies given ivermectin orally. *American Journal of Veterinary Research* **48**:684–685.

18 Hsu WH, Schaffer DD (1988). Effects of topical application of amitraz on plasma glucose and insulin concentrations in dogs. *American Journal of Veterinary Research* **49**:130–131.

19 Medleau L, Willemse T (1995). Efficacy of daily amitraz on generalised demodicosis in dogs. *Journal of Small Animal Practice* **36**:3–6.

20 Hugnet C, Buronfosse F, Pineau X, Cadoré J-L, Lorgue G, Berny PJ (1996). Toxicity and kinetics of amitraz. *American Journal of Veterinary Research* **57**:1506–1510.

21 White SD (1992). Otitis externa. *Waltham Focus* **2**:2–9.

22 Knottenbelt MK (1994). Chronic otitis externa due to *Demodex canis* in a Tibetan Spaniel. *Veterinary Record* **135**:409–410.

23 Folz SD, Ash KA, Conder GA, Rector DL (1986). Amitraz: a tick and flea repellent and tick detachment drug. *Journal of Veterinary Pharmacology and Therapeutics* **9**:150–156.

24 Cooper PR, Penaliggon EJ (1996). Use of fipronil to eliminate recurrent infestation by *Trichodectes canis* in a pack of Bloodhounds. *Veterinary Record* **139**:95.

25 Famose F (1995). Efficacy of fipronil (Frontline) spray in the prevention of natural infestation by *Trombicula autumnalis* in dogs. *Proceedings of The Royal Veterinary College Seminar: Ectoparasites and Their Control*, pp. 28–30.

26 Hunter JS, Keister DM, Jeannin P (1996). A comparison of the tick control efficacy of Frontline Spray against the American dog tick and brown dog tick. *Proceedings of the 41st Annual Meeting of the American Association of Veterinary Parasitologists*, Louisville, p. 51.

27 Curtis CF (1996). Use of 0.25% fipronil spray to treat sarcoptic mange in a litter of five-week-old puppies. *Veterinary Record* **139**:43–44.

28 Novotny MJ, Krautmann MJ, Ehrhart J, *et al.* (1999) Clinical safety of selamectin in dogs. *Proceedings of the American Association of Veterinary Parasitology*. New Orleans, p. 61.

29 McTier TL, McCall JW, Jernigan AD, *et al.* (1998) Efficacy of UK-124, 114, a novel avermectin for the prevention of heartworms in dogs and cats. *Recent Advances in Heartworm Disease Symposium*, Tampa, pp. 187–192.

30 Wren JA, McTier TL, Thomas CA, Bowman DD, Jernigan AD (1999). Efficacy of selamectin against *Toxacara canis* in dogs. *Proceedings of the American Association of Veterinary Parasitology*, New Orleans, p. 60.

31 Griffin CE, DeBoer DJ (2001). The ACVD task force on canine atopic dermatitis (XIV): clinical manifestations of canine atopic dermatitis. *Veterinary Immunology and Immunopathology* **81**:255–269.

32 Rosser EJ (2004). Causes of otitis externa. *Veterinary Clinics of North America Small Animal Practice* **34**:459–468.

33 Stogdale L, Bomzom L, van den Berg PB (1982). Food allergy in cats. *Journal of the American Animal Hospital Association* **18**:188–194.

34 Rosser EJ (1993). Food allergy in the cat: a prospective study of 13 cats. In: Ihrke PJ, Mason IS, White SD (eds). *Advances in Veterinary Dermatology, Volume 2*. Pergamon Press, Oxford, pp. 33–39.

35 White SD, Sequoia D (1989). Food hypersensitivity in cats: 14 cases (1982–1987). *Journal of the American Veterinary Medical Association* **194**:692–695.

36   Wills JM, Harvey RG (1994). Diagnosis and management of food allergy and intolerance in dogs and cats. *Australian Veterinary Journal* **71**:322–326.

37   Griffin CE (1993). Otitis externa. In: Griffin CE, Kwochka KW, Macdonald JM (eds). *Current Veterinary Dermatology*. Mosby, St Louis, pp. 245–262.

38   Maudlin EA, Ness TA, Goldschmidt MH (2007). Proliferative and necrotizing otitis externa in four cats. *Veterinary Dermatology* **18**:370–376.

39   Vidèmont E, Pin D (2010). Proliferative and necrotizing otitis in a kitten: first demonstration of T cell-mediated apoptosis. *Journal of Small Animal Practice* **51**:599–603.

40   Bond R, Anthony RM, Dodd M, Lloyd DH (1996). Isolation of *Malassezia sympodialis* from feline skin. *Journal of Medical and Veterinary Mycology* **34**:145–147.

41   Lorenzini R, Mercantini R, De Bernardis F (1985). *In vitro* sensitivity of *Malassezia* spp. to various antimycotic drugs. *Drugs Experimental Clinical Research* **11**:393–395.

42   Gupta AK, Kohli Y, Li A, Faergemann J, Summerbell RC (2000). *In vitro* susceptibility to the seven *Malassezia* species to ketoconazole, voriconazole, intraconazole and terbinafine. *British Journal of Dermatology* **142**:758–765.

43   Morris DO (1999). *Malassezia* dermatitis and otitis. *Veterinary Clinics of North America Small Animal Practice* **29**:1303–1310.

44   Morris DO (2004). Medical therapy of otitis externa and otitis media. *Veterinary Clinics of North America Small Animal Practice* **34**:541–555.

45   Strain GM, Merchant SR, Neer TH, Tedford BL (1995). Ototoxicity assessment of a gentamicin sulphate otic preparation in dogs. *American Journal of Veterinary Research* **56**:532–538.

46   Carlotti DN, Guaguere E, Denerolle P, Madin F, Collet JP, Leroy S (1995). A retrospective study of otitis externa in dogs. *Proceedings of the 11th Annual Meeting of the AAVD/ACVD*, Santa Fe, p. 84.

47   Paterson S, Payne L (2008). Brainstem auditory evoked responses in 37 dogs with otitis media before and after topical therapy. *Veterinary Dermatology* **19**:S30.

48   Kiss G, Radvanyi S, Szigeti G (1997). New combination for the therapy of canine otitis externa. I: Microbiology of otitis externa. *Journal of Small Animal Practice* **38**:51–56.

49   Mathison PT, Simpson B, Heithamer T, McCurdy D, Fadok V (1995). Development of a canine model for *Pseudomonas* otitis externa. *Proceedings of the 11th Annual Meeting of the AAVD/ACVD*, Santa Fe, p. 21.

50   Fraser G (1961). Factors predisposing to canine external otitis. *Veterinary Record* **73**:55–58.

51   Nuttall T, Cole LK (2007). Evidence-based veterinary dermatology: a systemic review of interventions for treatment of *Pseudomonas* otitis in dogs. *Veterinary Dermatology* **18**:69–77.

52   Ghibaudo G, Cornegliani L, Martino P (2004). Evaluation of the *in vivo* effects of Tris EDTA and chlorhexidine digluconate 0.15% solution in chronic bacterial otitis: 11 cases. *Veterinary Dermatology* **15**:65–67.

53   Yuan D, Shen V (1975). Stability of ribosomal and transfer ribonucleic acid in *Escherichia coli* B/V after treatment with ethylene-diamine tetra-acetic acid and rifampin. *Journal of Bacteriology* **122**:425–432.

54   Farca AM, Piromalli G, Maffei F, Re G (1997). Potentiating effects of EDTA-tris on the activity of antibiotics against resistant bacteria associated with otitis, dermatitis and cystitis. *Journal of Small Animal Practice* **38**:243–245.

55   Bogaard van den AEJM, Bohm ROB (1986). Silbersulfadiazincreme als therapie bei chronischen Pseudomonas infektionen des ausseren Gehorganges des hundes. *Prakt Tierarztl* **67**:971–980.

56   Noxon JO, Kinyon JM, Murphy DP (1997). Minimum inhibitory concentration of silver sulfadiazine on *Pseudomonas aeruginosa* and *Staphylococcus intermedius* isolates from the ears of dogs with otitis externa. *Proceedings of the 13th Annual Meeting of the AAVD/ACVD*, Nashville, pp. 12–13.

57 Foster AP, DeBoer DJ (1998). The role of *Pseudomonas* in canine ear disease. *Compendium on Continuing Education* **20**:909–919.

58 Kulick MI, Wong R, Okarma TB, Falces E, Berkowitz RL (1985). Prospective study of side effects associated with the use of silver sulphadiazine in severely burned patients. *Annals of Plastic Surgery* **14**:407–409.

59 Little CJL (1996). Medical treatment of otitis externa in the dog and cat. *In Practice* **18**:66–71.

60 Waker RD, Stein GE, Hauptman JG, MacDonald KH (1992). Pharmacokinetic evaluation of enrofloxacin administered orally to healthy dogs. *American Journal of Veterinary Research* **12**:2315–2319.

61 McKellar QA (1996). Clinical relevance of the pharmacological properties of fluoroquinolones. *Proceedings of the 2nd International Veterinary Symposium on Fluoroquinolones*, pp. 14–21.

62 Paterson S (2012). *Pseudomonas* otitis infection. *Clinician on call NAVC Clinician's Brief*. September pp. 59–64.

63 Metry CA, Maddox CW, Dirikolu L, Johnson YJ, Campbell KL (2012). Determination of enrofloxacin stability and *in vitro* efficacy against *Staphylococcus pseudintermedius* and *Pseudomonas aeroginosa* in four ear cleaner solutions over a 28 day period. *Veterinary Dermatology* **23**:23–26.

64 Salyer AA, Whitt DD (1994). *Pseudomonas aeuroginosa*. In: Salyers AA, Whitt DD (eds). *Bacterial Pathogenesis: a Molecular Approach*. ASM Press, Washington, pp. 260–270.

65 Nuttall TJ (1998). Use of ticarcillin in the management of canine otitis externa complicated by *Pseudomonas aeruginosa*. *Journal of Small Animal Practice* **39**:165–168.

66 Foster AP, DeBoer DJ (1998). The role of *Pseudomonas* in canine ear disease. *Compendium on Continuing Education* **20**:909–919.

CHAPTER 6 OTITIS MEDIA

1 Neer TM (1982). Otitis media. *Compendium on Continuing Education* **4**:410–417.

2 Cole LK, Kwochka KW, Kowalski JJ, Hillier A (1998). Microbial flora and antimicrobial susceptibility patterns of isolated pathogens from the horizontal ear canal and middle ear in dogs with otitis media. *Journal of the American Veterinary Medical Association* **212**:534–538.

3 Little CJL, Lane JG, Pearson GR (1991). Inflammatory middle ear disease of the dog: the pathology of otitis media. *Veterinary Record* **128**:293–296.

4 Bluestone CD, Doyle WJ (1988). Anatomy and physiology of the eustachian tube and middle ear related to otitis media. *Journal of Allergy and Clinical Immunology* **81**:997–1003.

5 Bluestone CD (1983). Eustachian tube function: physiology, pathophysiology, and role of allergy in pathogenesis of otitis media. *Journal of Allergy and Clinical Immunology* **72**:242–251.

6 Matsuda H, Tojo M, Fukui K, Imori T, Baba E (1984). The aerobic bacterial flora of the middle and external ears in normal dogs. *Journal of Small Animal Practice* **25**:269–274.

7 Little CJL, Lane JG, Gibbs C, Pearson GR (1991). Inflammatory middle ear disease in the dog: the clinical and pathological features of cholesteatoma, a complication of otitis media. *Veterinary Record* **128**:319–322.

8 Spreull JSA (1964). Treatment of otitis media. *Journal of Small Animal Practice* **5**:107–152.

9 Bruyette DS, Lorenz MD (1993). Otitis externa and otitis media: diagnostic and medical aspects. *Seminars in Veterinary Medicine and Surgery (Small Animal)* **8**:3–9.

10 Parker AJ, Chrisman CL (1995). How do I treat? Otitis media-interna in dogs and cats. *Progress in Veterinary Neurology* **6**:39–141.

11 Little CJL, Lane JG (1989). An evaluation of tympanometry, otoscopy and palpation for assessment of the canine tympanic membrane. *Veterinary Record* **124**:5–8.

12   Rose WR (1977). Surgery I: Myringotomy. *Veterinary Medicine/Small Animal Clinician* **72**:1646–1650.

13   Cox CL, Slack RWT, Cox GR (1989). Insertion of a transtympanic ventilation tube for the treatment of otitis media with effusion. *Journal of Small Animal Practice* **30**:517–519.

14   Remedios AM, Fowler JD, Pharr JW (1991). A comparison of radiographic versus surgical diagnosis of otitis media. *Journal of the American Animal Hospital Association* **27**:183–188.

15   Love NE, Kramer RW, Spodnick GJ, Thrall DE (1995). Radiographic and computed tomographic evaluation of otitis media. *Veterinary Radiology and Ultrasound* **36**:375–379.

16   Smeak DD, Crocker CB, Birchard SJ (1996). Treatment of otitis media that developed after total ear canal ablation and lateral bulla osteotomy in dogs: nine cases (1986–1994). *Journal of the American Veterinary Medical Association* **209**:937–942.

17   Trower ND, Gregory SP, Renfrew H, Lamb CR (1998). Evaluation of the canine tympanic membrane by positive contrast ear canalography. *Veterinary Record* **123**:78–81.

18   Hoskinson JJ (1993). Imaging techniques in the diagnosis of middle ear disease. *Seminars in Veterinary Medicine* **8**:10–16.

19   Hendee WR, Morgan CJ (1984). Magnetic resonance imaging. Part 1: Physical principles (medical progress). *Western Journal of Medicine* **141**:491–500.

20   Scherzinger AL, Hendee WR (1985). Basic principles of magnetic resonance imaging: an update. *Western Journal of Medicine* **143**:782–792.

21   Westersson P-L, Katzberg RW, Tallents RH, Sanchez-Woodworth RE, Svensson SA (1987). CT and MRI of the temporomandibular joint: comparison with autopsy specimens. *American Journal of Radiology* **148**:1165–1171.

22   Dvir E, Kirberger RM, Terblanche AG (2000). Magnetic resonance imaging of otitis media in a dog. *Veterinary Radiology and Ultrasound* **41**:46–49.

23   Chan KH, Swarts D, Doyle WJ, Wolf GL (1991). Assessment of middle ear status during experimental otitis media using magnetic resonance imaging. *Archives of Otolaryngology, Head and Neck Surgery* **117**:91–95.

24   Grandis JR, Curtin IN, Yu VL (1995). Necrotizing (malignant) external otitis: prospective comparison of CT and MR imaging in diagnosis and follow up. *Radiology* **196**:499–504.

25   Assoun J, Richardi G, Railhac J-J, *et al.* (1994). Osteoid osteosarcoma: MRI imaging versus CT. *Radiology* **191**:217–223.

26   Paterson S, Payne L (2008). Brain stem evoked auditory responses in 37 dogs with otitis media before and after topical therapy. *Veterinary Dermatology* **19**:S30.

27   Mansfield PD, Steiss JE, Boosinger TR, Marshall AE (1997). The effects of four commercial ceruminolytic agents on the middle ear. *Journal of the American Animal Hospital Association* **33**:479–486.

28   Igarashi Y, Suzuki J (1985). Cochlear ototoxicity of chlorhexidine gluconate in cats. *Archives of Otorhinolaryngology* **242**:167–176.

29   Igarashi Y, Oka Y (1988). Vestibular ototoxicity following intratympanic application of chlorhexidine gluconate in cats. *Archives of Otorhinolaryngology* **245**:210–217.

30   Igarashi Y, Oka Y (1988). Mucosal injuries following intratympanic application of chlorhexidine gluconate in cats. *Archives of Otorhinolaryngology* **245**:273–278.

31   Mansfield PD, Miller SC (2000). Ototoxicity of topical preparations. In: Gotthelf LN (ed). *Small Animal Ear Diseases: An Illustrated Guide*. Saunders, Philadelphia, pp. 145–154.

32   Strain GM, Merchant SR, Neer TM, Tedford BL (1995). Ototoxicity assessment of gentamicin sulphate otic preparation in dogs. *American Journal of Veterinary Research* **56**:532–538.

33 Gotthelf LN (2005). Diagnosis and treatment of otitis media In: Gotthelf LN (ed). *Small Animal Ear Diseases: An Illustrated Guide*, 2nd edn. Saunders, Philadelphia, pp. 275–303.

34 Anderson DM, White RAS, Robinson RK (2000). Management of inflammatory polyps in 37 cats. *Veterinary Record* **147**:684–687.

CHAPTER 7 OTOTOXICITY AND OTHER SIDE-EFFECTS OF OTIC MEDICATION

1 Merchant SR (1994). Ototoxicity. *Veterinary Clinics of North America* **24**:971–980.

2 Merchant SR, Neer TM, Tedford BL, Tewdt AC, Cheramie OM, Strain GM (1995). Ototoxicity of a chlorhexidine otic preparation in dogs. *Progress in Veterinary Neurology* **4**:72–75.

3 Aursnes J (1981). Vestibular damage from chlorhexidine in guinea pigs. *Acta Otolaryngologica* **92**:89–100.

4 Aursnes J (1981). Cochlear damage from chlorhexidine in guinea pigs. *Acta Otolaryngologica* **92**:259–271.

5 Mansfield PD, Steiss JE, Boosinger TR, Marshall AE (1997). The effects of four commercial ceruminolytics on the middle ear. *Journal of the American Animal Hospital Association* **33**:479–486.

6 Monkhouse WS, Moran P, Freedman A (1988). The histological effects on the guinea pig external ear of several constituents of commonly used aural preparations. *Clinical Otolaryngology* **13**:121–131.

7 Rosychuck RAW (1994). Management of otitis externa. *Veterinary Clinics of North America* **24**:921–951.

8 Morozono T (1988). Ototopical agents: ototoxicity in animal studies. *Annals of Otorhinolaryngology* **97**:S28–30.

9 Little CJL, Lane JG, Gibbs C, Pearson GR (1991). Inflammatory middle ear disease in the dog: the clinical and pathological features of cholesteatoma, a complication of otitis media. *Veterinary Record* **128**:319–322.

10 Ozkul A, Gedikogula G, Turan E (1998). Effect of intratympanic steroid application on the development of experimental cholesteatoma. *Laryngoscope* **108**:543–547.

11 Mansfield PD (1990). Ototoxicity in dogs and cats. *Compendium on Continuing Education* **12**:331–337.

12 Pickrell JA, Oehme FW, Cash WC (1993). Ototoxicity in dogs and cats. *Seminars in Veterinary Medicine and Surgery (Small Animal)* **8**:42–48.

13 Goycoolea MM, Paparella MM, Goldberg B, *et al.* (1980). Permeability of the round window membrane in otitis media. *Archives of Otolaryngology* **106**:430–433.

14 Goycoolea MV, Lundman L (1997). Round window membrane. Structure function and permeability: a review. *Microscopy Research and Technique* **36**:201–211.

15 Morizono T (1990). Toxicity of ototopical drugs: animal modelling. *Annals of Otolaryngology, Rhinology and Laryngology* **99**:42–45.

16 Hu DN, Qui WQ, Wu BT, *et al.* (1991). Genetic aspects of antibiotic induced deafness: mitochondrial inheritance. *Journal of Medical Genetics* **28**:79–83.

17 Gallé HG, Venker van Haagen AJ (1986). Ototoxicity of the antiseptic combination chlorhexidine/cetrimide (Savlon®): effects on equilibrium and hearing. *Veterinary Quarterly* **8**:56–60.

18 Igarashi Y, Suzuki J (1985). Cochlear ototoxicity of chlorhexidine gluconate in cats. *Archives of Otorhinolaryngology* **242**:167–176.

19 Igashi Y, Oka Y (1988). Vestibular ototoxicity following intratympanic application of chlorhexidine gluconate in the cat. *Archives of Otorhinolaryngology* **245**:210–217.

20 Igarashi Y, Oka Y (1988). Mucosal injuries following intratympanic application of chlorhexidine gluconate in cats. *Archives of Otorhinolaryngology* **245**:273–278.

21 Paterson S, Payne L (2008). Brain stem evoked auditory responses in 37 dogs with otitis media before and after topical therapy. *Veterinary Dermatology* **19**: S30.

22 Morizono T, Sikora MA (1982). The ototoxicity of topically applied povidone-iodine products. *Archives of Otolaryngology* **108**:210–213.

23 Aursnes J (1982). Ototoxic effect of iodine disinfectants. *Acta Otolaryngolica* **93**:219–226.

24 Merchant SR (1994). Ototoxicity. *Veterinary Clinics of North America Small Animal Practice* **24**:971–980.

25 Rosychuck RAW (1994). Management of otitis externa. *Veterinary Clinics of North America Small Animal Practice* **24**:921–952.

26 Griffin CE (1993). Otitis externa. In: Griffin CE, Kwochka KW, Macdonald JR (eds). *Current Veterinary Dermatology*. Mosby, St Louis, pp. 245–262.

27 Kiss G, Radvanyi S, Szigeti G (1997). New combination for the therapy of canine otitis externa. I: Microbiology of otitis externa. *Journal of Small Animal Practice* **38**:51–56.

28 Foster AP, DeBoer DJ (1998). The role of *Pseudomonas* in canine ear disease. *Compendium on Continuing Education* **20**:909–919.

29 Farca AM, Piromalli G, Maffei F, Re G (1997). Potentiating effects of EDTA-tris on the activity of antibiotics against resistant bacteria associated with otitis, dermatitis and cystitis. *Journal of Small Animal Practice* **38**:243–245.

30 Morais D, Gonzalez M, del Villar R, Gayoso MJ (1988). Long term ototoxic effects of neomycin applied topically in the middle ear – a morphological study in the guinea pig. *Journal of Laryngology and Otolology* **102**:304–307.

31 Kalkandelen S (2002). Comparative cochlear toxicities of streptomycin, gentamicin, amikacin and netilmicin in guinea-pigs. *Journal of International Medical Research* **30**:406–412.

32 Chen JM, Kakigi A, Hirakawa H, Mount RJ, Harrison RV (1999). Middle ear installation of gentamicin and streptomycin in chinchillas: morphologic appraisal of selective ototoxicity. *Journal of Otolaryngology* **28**:121–128.

33 Strain GM, Merchant SR, Neer TH, Tedford BL (1995). Ototoxicity assessment of a gentamicin sulphate otic preparation in dogs. *American Journal of Veterinary Research* **56**:532–538.

34 Mansfield PD, Miller SC (2000). Ototoxicity of topical preparations. In: Gotthelf LN (ed). *Small Animal Ear Diseases: An Illustrated Guide*. Saunders, Philadelphia, pp. 145–154.

35 Gotthelf LN (2005). Diagnosis and treatment of otitis media. In: Gotthelf LN (ed). *Small Animal Ear Diseases: An Illustrated Guide*, 2nd edn. Saunders, Philadelphia, pp. 275–303.

36 Ikiz AO (1999). An investigation of topical ciprofloxacin ototoxicity in guinea pigs. *Acta Otolaryngolica* **118**:808–812.

37 Moriello KA, Fehrer-Sawyer SL, Meyer DJ, Feder B (1988). Adrenocortical suppression associated with topical otic administration of glucocorticoids in dogs. *Journal of the American Veterinary Medical Association* **193**:329–331.

38 Green KM, Lappin DW, Curley JW, de Carpentier JP (1997). Systemic absorption of gentamycin ear drops. *Journal of Otolaryngology* **111**:960–962.

39 Weinstein MJ, Oden EM, Zeman WV, Wagman GH (1965). Antibiotic absorption after otic administration in dogs. *Antimicrobial Agents and Chemotherapy* **5**:239–244.

40 Gookin JL, Riviere JE, Gilger BC (1999). Acute renal failure in four cats treated with paromomycin. *Journal of the American Veterinary Medical Association* **215**:1821–1823.

41 Oishi N, Talaska AE, Schacht J (2012). Ototoxicity in dogs and cats. *Veterinary Clinics of North America Small Animal Practice*. **42**:1259–1271.

CHAPTER 8 AURAL ABLATION AND BULLA OSTEOTOMY

1 Layton CE (1993). The role of lateral wall resection in managing chronic otitis externa. *Seminars in Veterinary Medicine and Surgery* **8**:24–29.

2   Smeak DD, Kerpsack SJ (1993). Total ear canal ablation and lateral bulla osteotomy for management of end-stage otitis. *Seminars in Veterinary Medicine and Surgery* **8**:30–41.

3   Fossum TW (1997). Surgery of the ear. In: Fossum TW (ed). *Small Animal Surgery*. Mosby, St Louis, pp. 153–178.

4   Little CJ, Lane JG (1989). An evaluation of tympanometry, otoscopy and palpation for assessment of the canine tympanic membrane. *Veterinary Record* **124**:5–8.

5   Hettlich BE, Boothe HW, Simpson RB, Dubose KA, Boothe DM, Carpenter M (2005). Effect of tympanic evacuation and flushing on microbial isolates during total ear canal ablation with lateral bulla osteotomy in dogs. *Journal of the American Veterinary Medical Association* **227**:748–755.

6   Lane JG, Watkins PE (1986). Para-aural sinus in the dog and cat. *Journal of Small Animal Practice* **27**:521–531.

7   Cole LK, Kwochka KW, Kowalski JJ, Hillier A (1998). Microbial flora and antimicrobial susceptibility patterns of isolated pathogens from the horizontal ear canal and middle ear in dogs with otitis media. *Journal of the American Veterinary Medical Association* **212**:534–538.

8   Remedios AM, Fowler JD, Pharr JW (1991). A comparison of radiographic versus surgical diagnosis of otitis media. *Journal of the American Animal Hospital Association* **27**:183–188.

9   Trower ND, Gregory SP, Renfrew H, Lamb CR (1998). Evaluation of the canine tympanic membrane by positive contrast ear canalography. *Veterinary Record* **142**:78–81.

10 Penrod JP, Coulter DB (1980). The diagnostic use of impedance audiometry in the dog. *Journal of the American Animal Hospital Association* **16**:941–948.

11 Neer TM (1982). Otitis media. *Compendium on Continuing Education* **4**:410–417.

12 Love NE, Kramer RW (1995). Radiographic and computed tomographic evaluation of otitis media in the dog. *Veterinary Radiography and Ultrasound* **36**:375–379.

13 Lane JG (1979). Canine aural surgery. *In Practice* **1**:5–11.

14 Krahwinkle DJ (1993). External ear canal. In: Slatter D (ed). *Textbook of Small Animal Surgery*, 2nd edn. WB Saunders, Philadelphia, pp. 1561–1567.

15 Harari J (1996). Ear. In: Harari J (ed). *Small Animal Surgery*. Williams and Wilkins, Baltimore, pp. 193–199.

16 Trevor PB, Martin RA (1993). Tympanic bulla osteotomy for treatment of middle ear disease in cats: 19 cases (1984–1991). *Journal of the American Veterinary Medical Association* **202**:123–128.

17 Lane JG, Little CJL (1986). Surgery of the canine external auditory meatus: a review of failures. *Journal of Small Animal Practice* **27**:247–254.

18 Bradley RL (1988). Surgical management of otitis externa. *Veterinary Clinics of North America* **15**:813–844.

19 McCarthy RJ, Caywood DD (1992). Vertical ear canal resection for end-stage otitis externa in dogs. *Journal of the American Animal Hospital Association* **28**:546–552.

20 Pohlman DDL (1981). A modified surgical approach to chronic otitis externa. *Veterinary Medicine Small Animal Clinician* **76**:334–335.

21 Tirgari M, Pinniger RS (1986). Pull-through technique for vertical canal ablation for treatment of otitis externa in dogs and cats. *Journal of Small Animal Practice* **27**:123–131.

22 Smeak DD (2011). Management of complications associated with total ear canal ablation and bulla osteotomy in dogs and cats. *Veterinary Clinics of North America Small Animal Practice* **41**:981–994.

23 Hobson HP (1988). Surgical management of advanced ear disease *Veterinary Clinics of North America Small Animal Practice* **18**:821–844.

24 Elkins AD, Hedlund CS, Hobson HP (1981). Surgical management of ossified ear canals in the canine. *Veterinary Surgery* **10**:163–168.

25 White RAS (1995). Total ear canal ablation in the dog and cat. *Waltham Focus* **5**:23–28.

26 Smeak DD, de Hoff WD (1986). Total ear canal ablation: clinical results in the dog and cat. *Veterinary Surgery* **15**:161–170.

27 Mason LK, Harvey CE, Orsher RJ (1988). Total ear canal ablation combined with lateral bulla osteotomy for end-stage otitis in dogs: results in 30 dogs. *Veterinary Surgery* **17**:263–268.

28 Love NE, Kramer RW, Spodnick GJ, Thrall DE (1995). Radiographic and computed tomographic evaluation of otitis media in the dog. *Veterinary Radiology and Ultrasound* **36**:375–379.

29 Sharp NJH (1990). Chronic otitis externa and otitis media treated by total ear canal ablation and ventral bulla osteotomy in 13 dogs. *Veterinary Surgery* **19**:162–166.

30 Matthiesen DT, Scavelli T (1990). Total ear canal ablation and lateral bulla osteotomy in 38 dogs. *Journal of the American Animal Hospital Association* **26**:257–267.

31 Krahwinkel DJ, Pardo AD, Sims MH, Bubb WJ (1989). Effect of ear ablation on auditory function as determined by brainstem auditory evoked response and subjective evaluation. *Veterinary Surgery* **18**:60.

32 Payne JT, Shell LG, Flora RM, Martin RA, Shires PK (1989). Hearing loss in dogs subjected to total ear canal ablation. *Veterinary Surgery* **18**:70.

33 Beckman SL, Henry WB, Cechner P (1990). Total ear canal ablation combining bulla osteotomy and curretage in dogs with chronic otitis externa and media. *Journal of the American Veterinary Medical Association* **196**:84–90.

34 Devitt CM, Seim HB, Willer R, McPherron M, Neely M (1997). Passive drainage versus primary closure after total ear canal ablation/lateral bulla osteotomy in dogs: 59 dogs (1985–1995). *Veterinary Surgery* **26**:210–216.

35 Spivack RE, Elkins AD, Moore GE, Lantz GC (2013). Postoperative complications following TECA-LBO in dog and cat. *Journal of the American Animal Hospital Association* **49**:160–168.

36 Krahwinkel DJ, Pardo AD, Sims MH, Bubb WJ (1993). Effect of total ablation of the external acoustic meatus and bulla osteotomy on auditory function in dogs. *Journal of the American Veterinary Medical Association* **202**:949–952.

37 Holt D, Brockman DJ (1996). Lateral exploration of fistulas developing after total canal ablations: 10 cases (1989–1993). *Journal of the American Animal Hospital Association* **32**:527–530.

38 Smeak DD, Crocker BS, Birchard SJ (1996). Treatment of recurrent otitis media that developed after total ear canal ablation and lateral bulla osteotomy in dogs: nine cases (1986–1994). *Journal of the American Veterinary Medical Association* **209**:937–942.

39 Barrett RE, Rathfon BL (1975). Lateral approach to bulla osteotomy. *Journal of the American Animal Hospital Association* **11**:203–205.

40 Boothe HW (1988). Surgical management of otitis media and otitis interna. *Veterinary Clinics of North America* **18**:901–911.

41 Boothe HW (1998). Ventral bulla osteotomy: dog and cat. In: Bojrab MJ (ed). *Current Techniques in Small Animal Surgery*, 4th edn. Williams and Wilkins, Baltimore, pp. 109–112.

42 Seim HB III (1993). Middle ear. In: Slatter D (ed). *Textbook of Small Animal Surgery*, 2nd edn. WB Saunders, Philadelphia, pp. 1568–1576.

43 Denny HR (1973). The results of surgical treatment of otitis media and interna in the dog. *Journal of Small Animal Practice* **14**:585–600.

44 McNutt GW, McCoy JH (1980). Bulla osteotomy in the dog. *Journal of the American Veterinary Medical Association* **77**:617–628.

45 Bacon NJ, Gilbert RL, Bostock DE, White RAS (2003). Total ear canal ablation in the cat: indications, morbidity and long-term survival. *Journal of Small Animal Practice* **44**:430–434.

46 Ader PL, Boothe HW (1979). Ventral bulla osteotomy in the cat. *Journal of the American Animal Hospital Association* **15**:757–762.